Working *with* Toxic Older Adults

A Guide to Coping with Difficult Elders

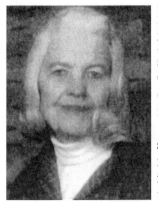

Moving from Minnesota to California following her marriage in 1948, **Gloria M. Davenport, PhD**, is still involved with aging activities after working in Orange County for 40 years, creating or developing a variety of programs in the helping professions.

Gloria received her BA and Pupil Personnel Counseling Credential at Chapman University, her MA in Social Science from California State University at Fullerton, a Certificate in Assertion Training at the University of California at Irvine, completed additional postgraduate work in Pastoral Counseling at Claremont School of Theology, and earned a PhD from Claremont Graduate University in Education in 1991 at the age of 63.

In 1972, as a professor at Santa Ana College, Gloria initiated, developed, chaired, and wrote the curriculum for a Human Services Department, being one of the first to incorporate training for older adult peer counseling. Subjects taught by Gloria were primarily in the areas of applied psychology and personal and professional growth and development. During the last 12 years of her tenure she was the Counselor for Reentry Students and Older Adults, teaching assertive self-development and personality-type classes. She retired in 1996 to complete her research for this book on toxicity in aging, a spinoff from her dissertation on "The Determinants of Successful Aging."

In 1992 Gloria originated a workshop and support-group program for adult children of toxic agers called ACTA. She has also presented at two American Society on Aging Conferences, and for 3 years wrote a monthly column on aging for the college's Older Adult Newsletter.

Gloria is a member of the American Society on Aging, the California Council on Gerontology and Geriatrics, The Association for Gerontology in Higher Education, the Orange County Behavioral Health Care—Older Adult Services Committee, and the Orange County Roundtable Aging Network. In 1982 and 1988 she received commendations for outstanding service to the elderly in Orange County.

She is also a member of the International Enneagram Association, the Association of Psychological Type, and for many years was a member of the International Transactional Analysis Association.

Working *with* Toxic Older Adults

A Guide to Coping with Difficult Elders

Gloria M. Davenport, PhD

with Foreword by Peggy Weatherspoon, MSG
Director, Orange County, California Area Agency on Aging

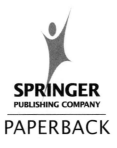

SPRINGER
PUBLISHING COMPANY

PAPERBACK

Springer Publishing Company, Inc.
11 West 42nd Street
New York, NY 10036

Cover design by Mimi Flow
Acquisitions Editor: Helvi Gold
Production Editor: Pamela Lankas

06 07 08 09 / 5 4 3 2 1

New ISBN 0-8261-0275-1 © 2006 by Springer Publishing Company, Inc.

Library of Congress Cataloging-in-Publication Data

Davenport, Gloria M.
  Working with toxic older adults : a guide to coping with difficult
elders / by Gloria M. Davenport.
            p   cm. — (Springer series on life styles and issues in aging)
        Includes bibliographical references and index.
        ISBN 0-8261-1223-4
        1. Aged—Psychology. 2. Aged—Care—Psychological aspects.
3. Aged—Family relationships—Psychological aspects.
4. Personality disorders. 5. Temperament. I. Title. II. Series.

HQ1061.D32 1999
305.26—dc21   98-45 133
                                                                        CIP

Printed in the United States of America by Bang Printing.

To all of you who live with,
work with,
associate with,
professionally serve,
teach about,
or want to prevent

Toxicity in Aging

Contents

Acknowledgments

One can never write a book without recognizing at least some of the individuals, concepts, values, and life experiences that stirred and percolated behind the book's unfolding.

I am no exception. I did, however, want to refrain from saying the proverbial, "without whom this book would never have been possible," but I don't see how I can avoid it. It's like growing old. One cannot do it well without the help and support of many people. Therefore, thanks. Thanks to all of you. I am deeply grateful.

Probably the greatest stimulant to this whole undertaking, the motivation for my interest in successful aging, or as I would prefer to call it, successful *living*, is someone I never thought I would be honoring—my mother. She, and also my father, were the epitome of a cliché I've come to respect: *"Pay attention to the person(s) who irritate or pain you the most. They are usually your mirror, and therefore, your best teacher(s)."*

Parents, along with spouses and children, are our best teachers. With me, unfortunately, it took 54 years and much self-imposed agony to discover this. The interaction may be positive or negative, conscious or unconscious. Regardless, the observation is constant. They model, we absorb. They talk, we watch and listen. The nonverbals are powerful. And we learn. *We choose.* We figure out what works. We write our own *script*, and we survive. Eventually we become strong enough to deal with whatever life hands us, that is, if we're open to its learning and willing to risk finding our Selves.

Then, we can *finally* say, "thank you" to our parent(s), even the toxic ones.

As for the others I want to thank, one learns very quickly family support is what really counts. Who but a loving spouse would read seemingly endless pages of manuscripts, sometimes three or four times because of countless rewrites, just to see if the words made sense to his logical mind. I hope if he understood them, you will also. Then those back rubs, plus fixing computer breakdowns, handling all the technical problems, and keeping the printer—and me—going? I'll be forever grateful, Hugh.

To Kim and Scott, our grown kids, their understanding and support for "whatever Mom's up to now" was valued. That included providing a cabin in Idaho, the first of three summers there, where I could write. Thanks Kim and Jally.

The lifetime of preparation, of self-discipline and studying, experiencing, teaching, and counseling that led to this book seemed as if a calling! There were people, workshops, conferences, classes, fieldwork, support groups, and theories: all critical to the outcome. I didn't say "thank you"; I just soaked it up.

Early in the book's inception, caring friends, like Gerry Starnes and Nancy Chase, critiqued the original manuscript. It was Gerry whose letter stimulated the first ACTA (Adult Children of Toxic Agers) workshop. What a great idea!

Others who helped in the early stages in a multitude of various ways were Joan Weiss Hollenbeck and her writing class; Jim Birren, PhD; Connie Goldman; Helena Malek; Brugh Joy, MD; Maria Estrada; Betty Goyne; Judy Reynolds; Joan Abrams; Peggy Weatherspoon; Vivian Stinson; Brenda Ross, PhD; Phil Dreyer, PhD; plus the many professionals who referred perceived toxic older adults for interviews.

Thanks also to Dorothy Nolte, PhD, who introduced me to Jerry Greenwald, PhD. It was Jerry who lent credence to my choice of the word "toxic." As far as I know he was the first to write on toxicity and nourishment in relationship patterns back in the late 1960s. His continuing support, encouragement, and friendship means much.

Naomi Feil, ACSW, is another professional whose acquaintance and support I honor. Her Validation Method and practical application with the maloriented old-old are a breakthrough in the gerontology field.

To the many professionals and service providers who shared their knowledge and experiences regarding toxic agers, my deepest gratitude. They are MarGreta Jorgensen, Janie Dam, Anh Nguyen, Burnie Hayes, Kathryn Wright, Rosemary Ford, Robert Cummings, Patricia Powers, Alyce Gratto, Linda Grant, Gail Smith, Lahoma Snyder, Shirley Lefkowitz, Sharon McNair, Wendy Klatzker, Jo Unger Wolf, Kathie Murtey, Jack Light, Charlene Edwards, Cordula Dick-Muehlke, PhD, Roseanne Kotzer, Bernice Byron, Jan Brady, Oscar Sandoval, Maureen Azeltine, Sharon Beard, Bud Taylor, Betsy Crimi, Rhonda Jarema, Connie Jones, Julio Rodriguez, and Gloria McDonough (Ortega). I just hope I did justice to their invaluable input.

Also, I'm deeply grateful to four special friends: Cheryl Svensson and Harry Moock for making time to read my later drafts and provide valuable feedback, Peggy Weatherspoon for her thoughtful Foreword and masterful critique and partial editing of the final draft, and Jim Birren for his support and willingness to also write a Foreword.

And to the editors and gerontology advisor at Springer publishing company, particularly Helvi Gold, the Acquisition Editor, a huge thanks. It was their inestimable wisdom, advice, encouragement, and guidelines that produced this final version.

Still, without the many unnamed caregivers, adult children, grandchildren, spouses, in-laws, and especially the "toxic agers" themselves who contributed so much this book would have been inconceivable. Their willingness to let me come into their lives at such a depth took courage. They allowed me to listen, to share their experiences, and to dig deep enough for doors to open to their repressed memories and emotional pain.

These were the individuals who made it possible to bring this anomaly of aging to light. To them (especially you T), I say THANKS. Thanks from the bottom of my heart. Because of them perhaps we, as a society, will no longer hide our heads in the sand regarding the small percentage (albeit a large number) of older adults who are not aging successfully. With this awareness, and a joint effort, it's realistic to believe that toxicity in aging can be prevented.

Foreword

Having known the author more than 20 years, I find Gloria Davenport to be one of the most positive and pleasant people I know, despite her own toxic familial relationships. Gloria is the real-life example of what she is revealing to us in her book—we can choose to be victims or we can choose to be triumphant. Having read her book, the maxim *"There are no victims—only volunteers!"* becomes reality. An important message in this work is that toxicity must not be tolerated by its intended victims.

This book is designed to help those who work with, know, and love toxic older persons. Through these pages we learn how to avoid the poison that toxic persons emit in many forms, thereby enabling us to continue to serve and love those who appear unlovable. To paraphrase one chapter, *It's not what I think of you that counts—it's what I think of my response to you.* The tools in this book teach us that if we know we are interacting with toxic persons we can manage our responses to them and avoid the psychological drain and emotional contaminants that lead to professional burn-out or personal despair.

The positive focus in this book on choice in lifestyles and adaptive social and spiritual behaviors offers hope and inspires us to continue with difficult work. For those of us who interact frequently with toxic older persons, and sometimes come face to face with our own demons in the process—this book demonstrates that balance and perspective are possible. Each of us has the power to change. It's never too late to learn and grow.

The chapter on personality theories helps us achieve greater understanding of toxic persons; the chapters on differential diagnosis are particularly helpful in demonstrating the complexities of the individuals and the many manifestations of toxic behavior. Gloria Davenport is clearly showing us that to be old and toxic is double jeopardy that begs creative solutions and challenges the best of us.

PEGGY WEATHERSPOON, MSG
Director, California Agency on Aging

Preface

People write books for many reasons. I'm writing because I cannot not do it.

Maybe it's because at age 70 writing a book for professionals in the gerontology field that will, I hope, also be read by adult children of toxic agers, caregivers, and older adults themselves might enable me to see a dream come true. Maybe, as expressed by Birren and Schaie in the Preface of their *Handbook of the Psychology of Aging* (1996), I too might be a stimulant that could lead "to improvement in the condition and quality of human life" if toxics, and those they touch, are helped to shift their perceptions and find the healing power of love deep inside themselves.

Maybe it's because, after what seemed like a lifetime of professional experience in the human-services and gerontology fields, I know how crucial it is to work with the whole person. Plus, there is that inner drive to share some of the things I have discovered in the last 10 years that might ease working with difficult older adults and uncover the hidden phenomenon of toxicity in aging.

How does one deal with the negative toxic energy and sense of victim consciousness particularly pervasive among self-reliant, independent-living, toxic agers?

For years I researched, worked with, made presentations, and wrote about toxicity in aging, plus facilitated workshop or support groups for adult children of toxic agers (ACTA). Then, after a presentation at the 1996 American Society on Aging Annual Conference, Springer Publishing asked if I would consider writing a book about toxic agers. It was the opening I needed. Here was a chance to integrate and present to other professionals what I had learned. It was a chance to crystallize my knowledge into a supplemental text that could be used as a resource for others.

One of my basic premises is that the still-prevalent negative stereotyping of aging and *gerontophobia** (Bunzel, 1972), and their opposites positive ageism and *gerontophilia* (Palmore, 1990, p. 39), are discrediting to the older adult and to a natural phase of life. My hope is for a realistic recognition that older adults come in all sizes, shapes, personalities, and temperaments. They, like all individuals, are unique and different. Some will be difficult. Some will be loving. Some will be toxic. Our task? To accept what they are and to deal with it.

Toxicity is *not* normal aging. Its symptoms are frustrating emotional stressors, confiscating valuable time and energy from social workers, therapists, caregivers, service providers, and those who must associate with a toxic ager, especially adult children.

This book is designed especially for professionals, service providers, and students in the gerontology field. It is also particularly pertinent to those of you who not only deliver services to toxic agers, but also happen to be an adult child of a toxic ager. Applying the book's content to your own self-assessment and personal or professional growth should be helpful.

In addition, this book is a practical guide for those of you who are adult children (often *co-Victims*) of toxic parents. The text will help you understand what is happening, learn how to block the passage of toxicity to the next generation, and bring forth your own resources.

If you are an older adult who simply wants to learn how to avoid the pitfalls of abnormal negativity in aging and to assess your own tendency toward toxicity, this book will give you some insights, intervention tips, and a self-assessment tool.

If you are middle-aged and a baby boomer beginning to think about your own aging process or if you just are curious about the

---

Note. Terms that are italicized (at first mention) are defined in the Glossary.

title, this book will provide some information about toxicity and its prevention.

To help meet these goals, the text has evolved into five parts. Part I uses definitions and descriptions to explain what is meant by toxic agers and whether it is a personality disorder as described in the *Diagnostic and Statistical Manual of Mental Health Disorders* (DSM-IV; American Psychiatric Association, 1994), why the focus on toxic agers, how we would know if we are toxic, and whether toxic agers are found in other ethnic groups. Part II looks at the impact of toxic agers on society, professionals, and co-Victims, and how this impact is handled. Part III examines how we become toxic, suggesting possible causes as adapted from other conceptualizations, theories, and models that can give us clues to this anomaly of aging. Part IV uses examples of intervention options plus proposes possible techniques and methods for professionals and adult children to intervene, cope, and uncover negative beliefs. Part V advocates following a spiritual path of unconditional love as the way to prevent toxicity and promote healing.

Research for this text was based on the premise, similar to Cohler's (1991), that when we're struggling to learn more about the drain of stressful events and relationships that cause daily hassles, studies must be closely tied to real-life situations. Consequently, most of the material on toxic agers was gained from personal contacts and in-depth interviews with more than 100 gerontology professionals and service providers who have toxic clients; with toxic older adults themselves and their adult children; and with spouses, grandchildren, in-laws, neighbors, and other professionals and from my personal, long-term counseling experience with a 76-year-old toxic college student, and my own mother. The rest of the information was obtained through related literature reviews, Feil's years of work with the maloriented, and Greenwald's multiple writings on toxicity and nourishment.

Pervasive throughout the following chapters is the hypothesis that *we respond to others and things according to the way we perceive them.* Expanded, this means that perception is projection. If we see someone as difficult, we will respond to him or her as if he or she is difficult. Likewise, if we perceive toxic agers as difficult, we will fear, avoid, challenge, or feel guilty when having to deal with them. We are not aware that these are our own perceptions, our own feelings and interpretations. We are not aware that it is our own "stuff," our own ego-defense mechanisms, projected onto the toxic ager. We use these defenses because we need them. They momentarily enable us to escape the fear and hurt inside and to avoid dealing with our own personal issues.

Toxics are not bad people; they *are* difficult. Not all difficult people are toxic, however, and not all toxics are old. Enforced (or voluntary) close proximity to adult children and multiple losses, such as control and dependency, may bring a lifelong toxicity to the surface. This *negative energy* is contagious for those susceptible to the *Victim consciousness* of older toxics. The goal for those working and associating with such agers is to learn how to protect and nourish themselves. Also, by blocking and shifting the projections that enable and maintain the syndrome, toxicity can be stifled or redirected.

Fortunately, the number of older adults who age unsuccessfully—and are locked into this anomaly—is proportionately small, but the impact on others is disproportionately vast. It is a behavior pattern that is little understood, isolated, and not acknowledged. To the public, it is a hidden syndrome.

By identifying this aging anomaly, labeling it to understand the pattern and what we are dealing with, working with possible causes rather than symptoms, proposing some strategies for coping, and suggesting ways to prevent its occurrence, it is hoped this Victim consciousness and negativity cycle can be interrupted before the baby boomers reach their late 70's.

In closing, it must be noted that toxicity is not a DSM-IV-certified personality disorder. It is a developmental character disorder and probably will be part of the new and growing field of character-oriented therapy. This means that the focus will be on an awareness of ego-controlled consciousness and a shift to move beyond the ego's defenses and unconscious compulsions toward healing, the reclaiming of true essence, and self-transformation.

With the above shift as the book's vision, one hopes it will be a catalyst for awakening readers to the premise that the task of aging is a spiritual journey, a journey wherein one finds his or her true self and wholeness.

List of Figures and Tables

Part I

What Do You Mean, Toxic?

We can protect ourselves from a poison only if it is clearly labeled as such.

—Alice Miller

Chapter 1

Introduction, Definitions, Descriptions

I called her "toxic."
John Steinbeck called her a "sad soul."
It could be someone you know.

I n his last book, *Travels with Charley—in Search of America* (pp. 46, 47), John Steinbeck wrote a description of a person he had met. It was a casual meeting, and only one encounter, but the impact was resounding:

> Strange how one person can saturate a room with vitality or excitement. Then there are others, and this dame was one of them, who can drain off energy and joy, can suck pleasure dry and get no sustenance from it. Such people spread a grayness in the air about them.
>
> I'd been driving a long time, and perhaps my energy was low and my resistance down. She got me. I felt so blue and miserable I wanted to crawl into a plastic cover and die.
>
> I went back to my clean little room. I don't ever drink alone. It's not much fun. And I don't think I am an alcoholic. But this night I got a bottle of vodka from my stores and took it to my cell. In the bathroom two water tumblers were sealed in cellophane sacks with

the words: "These glasses are sterilized for your protection." Everyone was protecting me and it was horrible. I tore the glasses from their cover. I violated the toilet seat with my foot. I poured half a tumbler of vodka and drank it and then another. Then I lay deep in hot water in the tub and I was utterly miserable and nothing was good anywhere.*

Two pages later, Steinbeck summarized it all:

A sad soul can kill you quicker, far quicker, than a germ. (p. 49)

That was 1962. Unfortunately, it's no different today. Sad souls are around us everywhere.

Although we have no clue as to the age of Steinbeck's character, it reveals that *toxicity* can emerge any time in adulthood. It appears that although toxic tendencies form in early childhood, the symptoms often remain covert unless an emotional trauma or severe loss foments the negative pattern.

With the onset of old age, however, when dependency and close proximity to adult children occurs, the invasiveness of toxicity surfaces. The behavior can no longer be hidden in acceptable, controlling roles or covered for by spouses.

Why the Term "Toxic Agers"?

In an emotional sense, what Steinbeck called "a sad soul" and I call a toxic ager personifies a psychosocial manifestation that can choke the spirit of anyone susceptible to its toxin. The destruction is slow, out of our awareness, and often goes unrecognized until the damage is done. Even gerontology professionals are not immune.

The affect of toxicity will range from simple annoyance to *frustration*, emotional entanglement and depression, withdrawal,

---

and thoughts of suicide. Professionals must watch for *countertransference.*

It was countertransference that caused me to label a group of unsuccessfully aging older adults, those I had interviewed for my dissertation on *Determinants of Successful Aging* (Davenport, 1991), as "*toxic.*" James Birren (personal communication, August 28, 1997) suggested that the label "noxious" might also be appropriate. Both terms imply that something is injurious to our health, with noxious expanding its effects to also mean harmful to our morals.

At the time of the interviews, I was attempting to learn why some elders aged so gracefully and others seemed to make it such a miserable journey. What was the difference? A blind study was designed in which subjects were preselected and matched in three categories: *very successful aging, successful aging,* and *unsuccessful aging* for comparison.

It took several 3- to 4-hour interviews with the unsuccessful agers before I realized that something was happening to my body. I began to pay attention. It felt as if I had been poisoned. It was then the term toxic flashed into my mind. Noxious just was not strong enough.

The difference between the interviews with the two groups of successful agers and the group of unsuccessful ones was striking. With the successful agers I felt exhilarated, stimulated, and comfortable. With the unsuccessful agers I felt professionally inadequate, depressed, anxious, totally drained of all my energy, and even angry and hurt. It happened consistently with every unsuccessful ager interviewed. The negativity and pattern of victimization were ever present. It always took 2 to 3 days for me to recover from each interview.

I dreaded every new encounter. My self-confidence was ebbing. What was going on? I had been in the helping professions for 40 years. I did not let clients get to me!

Puzzled, I rationalized that I was now in a different role. I was only a researcher, simply listening, soaking up the data and internalizing it, thoughtless of the need to protect myself. That satisfied me for about 6 months.

Then the day came when I could deny the truth no longer. With every toxic ager I interviewed, I was unconsciously returning to negative experiences with my own parents. I had lost my professional objectivity. I was forced to recognize and own a countertransference.

All wounds between my mother and myself had not healed as I had thought. They were simply buried and avoided. That worked for awhile. Now, however, unresolved personal emotions were interfering with my effectiveness as a professional. I felt ashamed. How could I be so unaware? So much in *denial?* So unprofessional?

The awakening only spurred me on. I had to learn more about this *anomaly* of *aging.* I arranged for a sabbatical and dug in. Despite my distaste for labels, the word "toxic" helped me to understand what I was dealing with and challenged me to conduct additional toxic-ager interviews with caring, objective nonattachment. My professional objectivity and effectiveness returned.

It was then I realized that this book had to be written. It is my hope that you will profit from my experience.

How Does Toxic Aging Compare with Successful Aging?

In my research on successful aging, I discovered a few comparisons with unsuccessful aging that might be helpful.

All subjects in the blind study were matched on culture, self-reliance, independent living, and a lack of mental or physical debilitations; were in the middle-income range; and were not experiencing grief. Subject ages ranged from 64 to 96, were both male and female and randomly selected from 168 referrals. Names were submitted to me by gerontology professionals, service providers, and others who worked with older adults in accord with the criteria established for each category.

Significant to me was the finding that although the *agers* who were successful had experiences and challenging illnesses similar to those of the unsuccessful agers, the successful elderly did not dwell on their ills. They faced them and got on with life. They assumed full responsibility for themselves, were problem solvers, had a positive attitude, maintained effective support systems, and did not play psychological *games.* With integrity, they were appropriately honest and direct with others.

The very successful agers were especially skilled at turning every negative situation into a positive one. The successful agers simply adapted, with ease, to whatever life offered them. Both groups learned from their experiences.

In contrast, the unsuccessful agers assumed no responsibility for their lives, solved few problems, and found fault with anyone they could not control or who tried to help (especially family). Nothing was ever right. Criticism and blame were the only responses. Negativity, self-centeredness, and victimization marked the emotional abuser's attitude. Only when the toxicity was severe enough to be publicly disruptive were social services engaged. Then they became the toxic ager's support system. Everyone else was disillusioned, feeling hopeless and bitter.

Definitions

To provide a common frame of reference for identifying toxic characteristics and behavior traits, the following definitions are offered. You are not asked to agree with them. You are only asked to use them as a basis for communication, clarity, and further understanding and exploration of toxicity in aging.

Toxic: According to the *Reader's Digest Great Encyclopedic Dictionary*, toxic means "pertaining to or caused by poison; poisonous."

If we liken this poison to a psychological toxin, we have a recognizable component that can also poison our mental, emotional, and physical systems, as well as produce its own antitoxin. This means that if we know what we are dealing with we can form a response pattern that keeps us immune to the poison.

Toxicity (Davenport's psychological definition): A *developmentally fixated* character maladaptation and life pattern of thinking, feeling, and perceiving that manifests in an obsessive negative energy of Victim consciousness and unaware controlling or compulsive behavior.

Some Explanations

According to Erikson, Erikson, and Kivnick (1986), the first stage of development is trust. Toxic agers do not achieve that level.

Fixated in distrust, they do not allow themselves the vulnerability of love (see chapter 9).

Toxicity is not a mental illness or a personality disorder as defined in the DSM-IV. (There is a more descriptive explanation found later in this chapter.)

Toxicity is the consequence of developmentally blocked, internally generated, fear-based choices and patterns of thinking, feeling, behaving, perceiving, and controlling that psychologically, socially, mentally, and spiritually poisons the self—and others that come in contact with the self—to the degree that those vulnerable to the toxic contamination may allow themselves to become co-Victims.

Toxicity in Agers: Manifests in pervasive negative behaviors and attitudes that have a destructive impact on social interactions. Such toxic behavior tends to alienate professionals, family, and friends, often leading to social isolation of the toxic person. In extreme cases, toxicity can lead to the withdrawal of services and social supports by the very individuals that the toxic ager needs for assistance in maintaining effective functioning or independent living, or both.

In a sense, toxics have an unconscious *addiction* to a false, ego-generated *self-perception* that they will be safe from their own repressed fears and *shadow* if they constantly maintain excessive control of themselves and others. Over time, however, this *perceptual process* becomes distorted, a rigidity sets in, standards are compulsively adhered to that are impossible to meet, self-righteousness rules, perspectives become unbalanced, and what could be their strengths of goodness and responsible power become their sources of weakness and downfall (see the discussion on the Enneagram, chapter 8).

Who Are Toxic Agers?

Toxic agers are older adults, usually in their 70's and 80's, who consistently act out defensive, negative behavior that is based on ego-distorted *perceptions*, values, beliefs, messages, and experiences. These perceptions are then projected onto others in varying degrees and levels of intensity and skill depending on the relationship and susceptibility of the other person to the toxic ager.

What Causes Toxicity?

No conclusive cause is evident at this time, but the exploratory, in-depth interviews conducted of toxic agers (Davenport, 1991) revealed that as children the feelings of toxic agers were not validated or allowed to be expressed. Submission to authority figures and blind obedience were the rule. Physical, verbal, emotional, and even sexual abuse were experienced. As a result, the abuse and restrictions modeled taught these older adults not to trust or love themselves, or others.

As children, these toxic agers were not allowed to feel, to ask for, or even know, what they needed. They did not understand that feelings were natural and could be appropriately and responsibly expressed. All they knew was that it was too vulnerable to feel, to love. They had to protect themselves from their environment. To certain personality types, this meant control, either overt demands or covert manipulations.

Does Extraversion or Introversion Make a Difference?

While reviewing the preceding description, a new insight emerged. Because toxicity manifests itself in various forms, it is logical that Jung's personality attitudes of *introversion* and *extraversion* are connected with the type of acting out, or in, exhibited by toxic agers (Jung, 1921).

In my original research I did not include this concept. Personal experience, however, affirms that the idea merits further study and could reveal another aspect of toxicity in agers.

For instance, in the initial study my personal reference to toxicity related only to my extraverted mother and her typical acting-out behavior. It did not occur to me until later that my father, an introvert, could also be toxic. His toxicity, as I have defined it, presented itself primarily in my childhood and precollege days, before I left home.

As an authoritarian, my father maintained a strong presence. Rules were rigid and strict and had to be obeyed immediately and without question or circumstance. Feelings were not granted expression. Orders and demands were expected to be fulfilled—perfectly. Yet, nothing was ever "right." He found fault with everything. As with my mother, pleasing him was impossible.

Because of a separation by distance, my father was old before I saw much of him again. He was withdrawn and rarely talked. I never knew what he was feeling. To him, silence meant strength. I now see it as an introvert's way of turning toxicity inward with aging.

What Is Toxic Behavior?

Toxicity is a pattern, a continuous, compulsive, and usually excessive acting out that induces a negative reaction and energy drain in anyone (especially professionals, caregivers, and adult children) who unconsciously and automatically "hooks" into (see Glossary) the toxic ager's psychological game bait and projections.

Low self-esteem, lack of trust, concealed fear, dependency, low self-confidence, and suppressed anger are some of the unconscious motivations for the highly honed *defense mechanisms* skillfully executed by toxics to protect their desperate, idealized, false image and *ego*. Defenses used are *acting out*, denial, *displacement, emotional insulation, help-rejecting, complaining, isolation of affects, projection* and *projective identification, rationalization, reaction formation,* and *rejection*.

Toxic behavior is generally identified by incessant and loud complaining, fault finding, whining, and blaming everyone else for problems. Defensively, all responsibility for the actions of toxic agers is thus removed. Toxics have no realization that their own choice of behavior is the cause of most of their difficulties.

This need to constantly control the environment is a driving force for most toxic agers. Rather than the more mature, internal locus of control displayed by successful agers, an external pattern of coping through suppression is typical of toxics, as reinforced by Ruth and Coleman (1996).

Because toxics know no other way to maintain their illusional need for certainty and personal power, they are usually insensitive, demanding, discounting, manipulative, attacking, critical, and well-known for the passive-aggressive guilt laid on loved ones. Pleasing or making toxic agers happy is impossible.

Is Toxicity Verbal Abuse?

Because verbal abuse is the most visible sign of toxicity, the unceasing negative thinking and projections of toxic agers are the focus here. Verbal abuse often leads to emotional damage that can systematically dismantle and undermine the self-esteem and confidence of anyone who must work with, serve, care for, or relate to toxics *if* they do not understand what they are dealing with or are personally susceptible to and internalize the psychological poison.

In her book *When You and Your Mother Can't Be Friends* (1990, p. 107), Secunda recounts the actions of a toxic ager as she describes "the Critic":

> The Critic is a woman in a state of constant dread, like a fugitive on the run—she is terrified someone will discover that she is really as unworthy as she accuses everyone else of being. The zeal with which she demeans her children is a desperate attempt to salvage, by comparison, some small shard of self-esteem. She conceals her tremulousness behind a wall of barbs, and digs, and nagging.

Unrealistic as this may appear, adult children of toxic parents, and even some professionals, are caught in the same defense-projection scenario. The more the helper gives, or the more he or she tries to please the toxic, the greater the demands and the denigration. Toxic agers do not know how to handle positive caring. Instead, they appear stuck, unable to break out of the increasingly hardened (if conceded) pattern of projected cover-up and control. In their deluded thinking, they believe that if they reveal their fears and weaknesses they will lose even the obligated connections they do have; they do not realize they are already destroying the very thing they need the most: the unconditional love and shared sense of emotional support from loved ones.

It is crucial for those of us who live, love, and work with toxic agers to be aware of the dysfunctional interplay between the toxic parent and the adult child. Avoidance can sabotage your time and effectiveness if it is not considered as part of the service (see chapters 5 and 6).

Working with toxicity at any age is frustrating, but the long-held, rigid patterns of toxic agers are particularly challenging. As confirmed by Patricia Evans (1996) in her book the *Verbally Abusive Relationship*, emotional and verbal abuse is usually hidden and kept secret within the family only to become more aggravating and troublesome over time.

Is Toxicity Emotional Blackmail?

Susan Forward, the author of *Toxic Parents* (1989), proposes in her new book (1997) that when people use Fear, Obligation, and Guilt to manipulate you, it is emotional blackmail. She calls it FOG, and that is exactly what an aged toxic parent will do to his or her adult children, or any geriatric service provider, if it is allowed.

In a sense, blackmail is easy for toxic agers because they have had years to develop an uncanny way of knowing every hot button to push in people they meet (Forward, 1997, p. 102). It leaves professionals or adult children feeling guilty if they believe they are obligated to meet every demand presented, even though it may be excessive and unrealistic. Watch for this tactic because it is particularly unnerving when a client threatens to go to your supervisor if his or her demands are not met.

Is Toxicity a Mental Illness?

During 8 years of research and teaching about toxic agers, I have resisted labeling toxicity as a mental illness. As primarily an educator, my bias is evident. Although toxicity is a form of personality disorder, I perceive it as a developmental problem, not psychopathology, as an educational issue, not a clinical one. How you perceive it is the key. It all depends on your interpretation and the need to operationalize a diagnosis for insurance purposes.

For most professionals, if the description is found in the American Psychiatric Association's (APA, 1994) *Diagnostic and Statistical Manual of Mental Disorders* (DSM-IV), it is a mental illness. At this point, the word "toxic" is not a label.

Gerontology researchers Gatz, Kasl-Godley, and Karel (1996) advise we be more cautious. They state that "the literature reviews and a small study of clinical reports suggest that none of the older patients sufficiently met the diagnostic criteria of a mental illness according to the DSM-III-R" (1987, edition preceding the DSM-IV) and that perhaps the "criteria for a personality disorder should be age-specific" (p. 373). They submit that there is a "need for different diagnostic categories or criteria to capture qualitative age differences." Otherwise, it is too easy to place older adults under the DSM category NOS, "Personality Disorder Not Otherwise Specified" (APA, 1994, p. 629), a catchall for all deviant behavior that does not match the specific DSM classifications.

Consequently, caution in applying DSM classifications is paramount. Although toxicity does not fit any of the 10 common, and specific, personality disorders, in its severest form, toxicity does sound like the DSM-IV description of a General Personality Disorder, which is described as "enduring patterns of inner experience and behavior that deviates markedly from the expectations of the individual's culture," and that the "perceiving, thinking, and relating . . . is inflexible and maladaptive" (APA, 1994, p. 630). Also, when older adults are in this stage of toxicity, they show, and cause, "significant functional impairment or subjective distress," as indicated in the criteria set forth in the "Diagnostic Features of a Personality Disorder" (APA, 1994, p. 630).

Jolting? Yes! But the key words here are "significant functional impairment" and "subjective" distress. Depending on the degree of toxicity, most toxics function well in public—they can even be charming if they so choose—and any "subjective distress" is usually unfelt because it is displaced on others, especially family.

Consequently, unless a thorough evaluation is made and maladaptive personality traits and a clinical personality disorder are clearly differentiated, misdiagnoses will occur because both tend to manifest themselves in "distorted ways of perceiving oneself or other people, including obliviousness to one's effect on others, and inappropriate responses" (Gatz et al., 1996, p. 373).

Notwithstanding the lack of pertinent diagnostic data regarding older adults, the APA does warn that "Although, by definition, a Personality Disorder requires an onset no later than early adulthood, individuals may not come to clinical attention until relatively late in life. A Personality Disorder may be exacerbated following the loss of significant supporting persons (e.g., a spouse) or previously stabilizing social situations (e.g., a job)" (APA, 1994, p. 631).

Nevertheless, obtaining the data necessary for differentiating the connection between clinical disorders and toxicity is difficult. Older adults of the Depression generation especially are not prone to share their emotional pain, voluntarily go to a mental health therapist, or have an accurate memory of early life experiences. Time and patience, and watching for nonverbal clues, are of the essence.

Just remember, when making an assessment of older adults, most toxicity never reaches "the threshold" of the specified diagnostic criteria for the DSM personality disorders or its "qualitatively distinct clinical syndromes" (APA, 1994, p. 633).

What About Multiple Diagnoses?

Multiple diagnoses are difficult enough to manage without adding toxicity to the mixture. Most professionals will attend first to the presenting problem(s), such as physical illness, alcoholism, dementia, and drug abuse only to discover that the toxicity, which may have been considered a secondary problem, ultimately becomes a major issue.

Toxic agers are usually not willing clients. Initially they will deny being told anything is wrong with them. If they are coerced or manipulated into seeing a professional, they will sabotage treatment within days by refusing to follow directions, resisting taking medication as prescribed, or supplementing medications with over-the-counter remedies or alcohol.

When a drinking pattern is involved, differentiation between early and late onset must be considered. Marilyn Milligan, a licensed clinical social worker (LCSW) and Behavioral Health Care, Older Adult Services Coordinator in Orange County, California, in a report on substance abuse among older adults, indicates that if the drinking pattern is early in onset, "delayed developmental coping strategies," such as possessed by toxic agers, make a "poor prognosis" (Milligan, 1997).

Agencies do recognize and consider the difficulties presented by toxics and plan and develop pilot programs accordingly. For example, Milligan's report on Orange County's Older Adult Substance Abuse Demonstration Project indicated that the criteria for program acceptance included "family involvement, being receptive to agency involvement, and any risk factor which would impact functioning" or the success of the endeavor (Milligan, 1997).

Regardless, each diagnosis must be made on a case-by-case basis, and should be flexible and open to the varying complications of each client. Toxicity, for instance, may worsen with dementia or, as in the case of my own mother, improve with dementia. With her, the negative discounts faded along with her memory.

What About Toxicity and Physical Challenges?

As with the other multiple diagnoses, toxicity just makes situations more difficult. In the case of the physically challenged, how the diagnosis is perceived is critical. Toxics tend to use it to enable their "learned dependency," unless they are in an agency that will not tolerate such "poor me" dependency.

According to one such agency's manager, Robert D. Cummings, Executive Director of a California independent living center,

> Our tolerance for toxicity is low because the agency's ultimate goal is independency, by people making their own choices. Like other disabilities, if toxics are not confronted, we only enable the continuance of the pattern, and thus allow others to be infected. We naturally do all we can to help, but only when the acting-out stops and a choice for life is made. (personal communication, February 25, 1998)

Although this agency had no older persons participating at the time of the interview, Cummings did give me an example of toxicity in a disabled older person that illustrated the problem of "learned dependency" and its repercussions. He told the story of a director friend from another agency who had a blind female in her mid- to late-70's on that agency's Board of Directors. "The experience was very hard on my friend," said Cummings, "because she didn't understand toxic behavior. Every time she tried to help the Board member, my friend was shot down and felt like a failure."

In response to offers of help, the senior volunteer would just continue her whining with tiresome vehemence and persistence. "I shouldn't be on the Board because I can't contribute to the meetings. I'm not able to read the material and minutes prior to each meeting."

After being told that the whole packet of material was recorded, the older woman refused to use the audiotapes, an indicator of toxicity and psychological game playing called "If It Weren't For . . . " and "Poor Me" (see chapter 10, the section on transactional analysis [TA]).

At Board meetings the older woman constantly interrupted, contradicted others in the discussions, asked pointless questions, and used her blindness as an excuse for her behavior. She was the Victim. It wasn't her fault; therefore, she wasn't responsible. At home, the woman refused to cook and insisted that Meals on Wheels be brought in but complained about the quality of service.

While Cummings described this scene, I detected a tone of disgust in his voice. Later I learned that he lives alone, does all his own cooking, runs one of the largest and best agencies for the disabled in California, and is on national boards, despite his own blindness, diabetes of 36 years, liver problems, dialysis for 1 1/2 years, and kidney transplant.

I also learned that part of the irritation was due to the fact that his friend, like so many well-meaning professionals, did not have the courage to confront or put boundaries around the toxic ager. Instead, the director waited until the ager's term of office was up, wrote the usual letter of thanks for the service, and enabled the pattern's continuance.

"People make their own choices," Cummings said, a philosophy that permeates his agency and its extensive staff training, including weekly time off for college classes on how to deal with the full dynamics of working with multiple complaints and diagnoses. With choices, people can "waste their lives, or make them come alive." The responsibility is theirs.

Is Toxicity Found in Other Ethnic Groups and Cultures?

Toxicity does occur in all cultures and ethnic groups, but it may be difficult to identify. Not all nonconforming minority behavior is toxic. Consequently, careful consideration is critical in differentiating social and ethnic customs, expressions, and values that may constitute behavior similar to what we judge as toxic.

Obtaining such information, however, took some time and patience because connections and trust were necessary before most of the minority-group representatives were willing to reveal anything negative about individuals in their own group. As they did, however, a plethora of examples and explanations came forth. So rich in humanness and understanding are these stories that chapter 2 is devoted to their portrayal.

How Are Toxic Agers Perceived?

In my follow-up research on toxic agers, I asked professionals, service providers, caregivers, spouses, and adult children involved with toxics on a daily basis to describe their perceptions of their experiences with these older adults. Some of the responses were as follows:

- Toxics are impossible to work with. They chase everyone away, even family.
- A toxic is a negative and self-centered person who exhausts and alienates anyone who wants to help.
- Toxics are more than difficult; they will destroy a group, program, or plan in seconds.
- Toxics complain incessantly. They always blame others for their problems.
- Toxics are immersed in self-pity and see themselves only as Victims.
- Toxicity is self-poisoning. It's a pattern of blaming, of destructive behavior.
- Toxicity is a conscious/unconscious refusal to deal with misunderstandings in personal relationships.
- Toxic people do not take responsibility for their lives. They manipulate others. And the more self-control they relinquish, the more they become blaming, vindictive, suspicious, hostile, critical, and eventually self-pitying and martyred.
- Toxicity may close areas of the brain or heart when the practice becomes habitual.

Summary

"Toxic agers" is the term used to describe a small percentage of older adults, usually in their late 70's and 80's, whose lifestyle and behavior make life miserable and difficult for anyone who takes in the psychological poison the toxics project on them.

In the context of this text, toxicity is defined as the negative energy of Victim consciousness that necessitates a psychosocial–spiritual approach to *healing*, not a cure. Behavioral descriptions are included in the definition, but the term "toxic agers" is used primarily to call attention to a developmentally fixated, *maladaptive* behavior that can destroy family relationships and leave the older adult lonely and unloved and the professional involved frustrated.

Toxic behavior is demeaning and manipulative and carries guilt-inducing, passive-aggressive comments and unreasonable demands. It is not a mental illness as described in the DSM-IV (APA, 1994), but it is a form of personality disorder that, when combined with other multiple afflictions, can impede treatment. The manifestation of toxicity will also vary, depending on whether the toxic person functions as an introvert or an extravert.

Toxicity is multiethnic and is found wherever human beings exist. Religious and physically challenged groups are no exception. How we respond to these groups, and the toxic agers within them, however, will differ in accord with our own values, customs, needs, understanding, culture, and projected and self-perceptions.

Therein lies the major hypothesis of this book. We respond to people and things according to the way we perceive them. If a negative condition, situation, or relationship is not understood, does not meet group expectations, or is guilt or fear generating, and thus disowned, it is projected onto an external object, person, or group. It is that projection—our own perception—to which we, and toxics, respond. Consequently, looking inside ourselves at our own internal conflicts, dynamics, and issues is the key to dealing with toxic agers and avoiding countertransference.

The following chapters will expand on the impact of toxicity on other ethnic and cultural groups, professionals, families, and other potential co-Victims. The need to understand an individual's background, beliefs, values, habits, relationships, and circumstances before labeling him or her as toxic is also depicted.

Although considered a long-term developmental issue, concealed toxicity can erupt when sudden trauma, drastic change, or severe losses, such as a job, spouse, independence, or self-image, remove an acceptable role cover and perceived sense of power and control. The *personality* becomes vulnerable and less adaptable when new and unfamiliar *stressors* exceed optimal levels of *stress*.

Chapter 2

Why the Focus on Toxic Agers?

Not all older adults are aging successfully. Toxicity is a major reason.

Raising Consciousness

Toxicity in agers is a psychosocial-spiritual anomaly of growing old, misunderstood by many, feared by some, and hidden from most except the families and gerontological service specialists who are forced to deal with it. Looking afresh at this disparity of aging is the focus of this book. Toxic agers have much to teach us all.

Can you imagine what it would be like to be an older person no one wants to be around, to feel alone and miserable? To have loved ones, friends, and even clergy rarely come to visit? To have service providers resist making a house call?

"I want to help her," they say. "I want to visit. I want to care about her, but I just can't handle the negativity, the demeaning attitude, the putdowns, and always being blamed for all her problems. I feel so frustrated, so helpless, and so resentful after all I've tried to do to help. I just can't deal with it . . . maybe I'm in the wrong profession!"

Facing Reality

No longer can we ignore this toxic anomaly of aging. The pattern is disturbing if one considers that it is passed on from one generation to the next unless interrupted. In 20 years the first of the baby boomers will be in their 70's, a staggering thought if we consider the ramifications. That is 75 million people. If even only 5% of them become visibly toxic, that is still 3.75 million people!

Can we awaken them to early intervention, to prevention? Can we model for the baby boomers what not to become?

If we multiply the baby boom number by the number of adult children and grandchildren who are being exposed to this syndrome and may have already adopted some of their elders' toxic thinking, traits, and behaviors, then add the impact on service providers, spouses, in-laws, neighbors, friends, relatives, and the taxpayer, the thought of the multiplied toxicity in society is frightening.

Is it possible things might be different with the baby boomers? Will they have enough self-love to choose to age successfully, to be self-nourishing, responsible, and whole or are their current self-centered, quick-fix expectations going to prevail?

We can pray there will be a change. The teaching role of the professional is all the more critical as we examine the demographic data projected for the future. Reversing the Victim consciousness trend and preventing the spread of toxicity to millions of future agers may be one of our greatest challenges.

A Look at the Demographics

Much of the following data has already been used in public policy planning and gerontological research. It is also vital for those of us who provide daily services to older populations. Informed awareness will enable us to understand and plan for the differences and uniqueness of future aging generations. Change is coming, and we as gerontology professionals especially need to be prepared. Geriatric services must not remain the same.

Population Projections

According to the pamphlet on American elderly issued in 1993 by the U.S. Department of Commerce, there were 3.1 million elderly in the United States in 1900, about 1 in 25 Americans. By 2020, the population is projected to be 54 million, or 1 in 6 Americans. By 2011, the first members of the baby boom will reach age 65; more children will know their great grandparents; and four generations in a family will be common. By 2050, during the final phase of the gerontological explosion, the number of elderly could reach 79 million, or about 1 in 5 (U.S. Commerce, 1993, pp. 2, 3).

These projections are based on the early 1990 trends in fertility, mortality, and immigration. It is assumed the trends will continue. If mortality decreases due to better health habits and medical advances, the number of elderly will be even higher (U.S. Commerce, 1993, p. 4).

Racial Group Projections

In 1990, Whites were the highest proportion of elderly of any racial group in America, primarily because they have higher survival rates and lower fertility rates. Immigration of Whites has also declined, meaning that by 2050, the White elderly population will be proportionally even larger (U.S. Commerce, 1993, p. 4).

On the other hand, other racial groups will also be expanding, yielding the most diverse population of elderly in U.S. history. For example, the Hispanic population of elderly, age 65 and up, was 1.1 million in 1990. It is projected to be 12 million by 2050, 11 times as many; the number of Hispanics 80 years and over will increase from about 200,000 in 1990 to more than 4.5 million in 2050 (U.S. Commerce, 1993, p. 5).

State Populations

In 1990, nine of the most populous states—California, Florida, New York, Pennsylvania, Texas, Illinois, Ohio, Michigan, and New Jersey—had more than 1 million elderly each. California has the largest number of elderly, but Florida has the nation's highest proportion of elderly, 18% (U.S. Commerce, 1993, p. 6).

The number of elderly increased in every state between 1980 and 1990, with the greatest increase in the western and southeastern coastal states.

Another high proportion of elderly (13%) is found in the midwestern states of North Dakota, South Dakota, Nebraska, and Iowa, primarily due to the migration out of the young.

Sex Distribution

About 1.3 million of the 1.6 million elderly living in nursing homes are female, and that number increases drastically with age. This is due largely to the longer life span of women, early widowhood, living alone longer, and becoming too frail to care for themselves. Chronic illnesses, disabilities, and dependency become the norm.

The implications of this decreasing sex ratio on the health, social, and economic problems of *old-old* women have long been known to gerontologists, but consideration for the psychological and spiritual challenges is sparse.

Household Changes

Because the aging are continuing to live longer, the poverty of many widowed women living alone is getting attention. Promotion has also been given to the popularly labeled "sandwich generation" and supportive time off from employment for physical care of disabled parents. Few professionals such as therapists, social workers, counselors, teachers, clergy, case managers, and professional caregivers, however, are specifically trained to work with the psychological and spiritual needs of toxic agers or to deal with the projections and psychological games they play with older adult children, families, communities, and professionals themselves. The deterioration of the relationship affects all and interferes with treatment.

Granted, the concept, or at least the label, of *toxicity in agers* is new, but its implications in the psychological field are not.

Need for Early Awareness of Toxicity

Gestalt therapist, group facilitator, professor, and author, Jerry Greenwald was the first (as far as I know) to postulate on the concepts of toxicity as it relates to adult behavior. His original monographs *The Art of Emotional Nourishment* (1968) and *The Art of Emotional Nourishment: Self-induced Nourishment and Toxicity* (1969) were the forerunners of his bestseller *Be The Person You Were Meant To Be: Antidotes to Toxic Living* (1973).

Although not focused specifically on the older adult, Greenwald's concepts and descriptions of toxicity are universal and applicable to any age, since toxicity is a lifelong pattern. Specific characteristics of toxicity will be described later in this chapter. The major difference is that toxicity gets more visible and troublesome as the years pass and proximity to adult children intensifies.

Shadow Work

According to my observations, instead of using their later life to accomplish its prescribed task of spiritual growth and wholeness, toxic agers are struggling with *integrity*. Their self-perceptions conflict and are laden with guilt, anxiety, imperfection, fear, and loss of control, or as Jungian psychologists would say, their suppressed shadow self. Hidden in the unconscious is the toxic ager's true *Self.* It is buried deep because its expression during the developmental years was perceived as a sin, thus intuitively deemed unsafe.

The shadow self is a life force that has never been trained, resists containment, and grows stronger with age. It will emerge unexpectedly, fearful only of exposure to light. Since it is disowned and forbidden, much effort is expended by toxic agers to control its potent energy and prevent the shadow from breaking through. Although it is suppressed and unrecognized, agers have learned to fear its expression and force. They sense something uncontrolled is operating inside them. Thus, the struggle to contain the shadow is ever present.

Ironically, the only thing that can help is self-love and nourishment, the one thing toxics are incapable of doing. They don't know how. They are unable to open up, trust, and be vulnerable enough to let go of the controls, to feel, to accept, and to embrace the healing power of spiritual love in order to become free and whole.

The strain of trying to be something they are not, of maintaining an ego illusion of power and safety, worsens as older adults age. Added to this is their increasing reliance on adult children while clinging to the perception that they are still in the strong, controlling parent role and must act accordingly.

Faulty Needs Patterns

The stress of trying to meet false psychological needs is intensified when toxic agers persistently refuse, or are unable, to honestly face, own, and appropriately communicate their true needs and feelings to professionals or to adult children. Unacknowledged, the toxics generally don't know what they feel or need or how to express it. As with unaccepted talents and desires, needs are also hidden shadow parts, lost to conscious awareness.

Relational problems are strained to the limit. Lack of skills needed to effectively meet these needs and the inability to experience intimacy are the key ingredients that separate toxics from nourishing people. Adult children, as well as some professionals, usually do not understand the dynamics or how to deal with it.

Consequently, they hook into the toxics' psychological games, only to perpetuate the toxicity and become co-Victims. Too often, professionals get caught in the middle, a time-consuming, futile trap, if we are not aware.

Horney's Inner Conflict Strategies

Greenwald was not the first to look at faulty personality patterns. Horney's (1945/1992) classic work on *neurosis* also speaks to the issue. Here it is clear that toxic agers have many of the same faulty needs issues as those Horney classified as neurotic. It is also clear that toxics and neurotics use very similar strategies to relieve these inner turmoils.

Three such strategies formulated by Horney (1945/1992, p. 17) are commonly found in toxics. They are revealed by displays of faulty perceptions and thinking and subsequent lack of social skills. The strategies are as follows:

- *Arbitrary rightness,* to quell inner doubts
- *Rigid self-control,* for holding themselves together by sheer will power
- *Cynicism,* to eliminate any internal conflict by discounting others' values

According to Horney "these conflicts can be resolved by changing the conditions within the personality that brought them into being . . . making them less fearful, less hostile, and less alienated from self and others" (1945/1992, p. 17).

More on Horney's Neurosis

To Horney, neurosis is a "disturbance of the personality and a source of psychic illness" (1945/1992, p. 11). It is not new. It was known to poets and philosophers of all times. Within each of us are driving, compulsive forces that we form into a character structure based on an idealized image. If our true nature conflicts with this image, there is a collision of values and expectations. Fearing the torment of the inner conflicts, we blind ourselves to the contradictions that tear us apart inside and bury the parts of ourselves we cannot tolerate, the shadow. The neurosis is then generated by the disturbances from within that are projected onto our relationships with others.

The key significance here is Horney's radical divergence from the traditional treatment. According to her premise, it then follows that the neurotic's (and toxic's) difficulties are not from past experiences "but depend rather upon understanding the interplay of forces in our existing personality." Therefore, "recognizing and changing ourselves with little or even no expert help is entirely feasible" (1945/1992, p. 14).

Nourishment Versus Toxicity

Greenwald (1969) proclaims that self-nourishment is the way to bring about the change in conditions within the personality to which Horney refers.

Each of us, according to Greenwald (1969), is fully responsible for our own nourishment and the kinds of relationships in which we involve ourselves. Whether these relationships are nourishing or toxigenic, the subsequent gratification or frustration is always our choice. Because we all have both nourishing and toxic qualities within us, it is our responsibility to generate the positive pattern. We can intrapsychically poison ourselves and extrapsychically poison others, or we can spread self-love and turn around a nation's Victim consciousness mind-set.

Lack of awareness of what we do to ourselves or lack of knowledge of how to change is no excuse. It does not remove the reality of the toxigenic process, a function of our unconscious shadow and lack of ego approval. Consequently, toxic agers are stuck with their negative patterns unless they wake up to what and who they are and are willing to expend the effort and discipline to change. For advanced toxics that effort is not likely.

Characteristics of Self-Induced Toxicity

The first step in transformation is the understanding of the characteristics of toxicity. With Greenwald's permission, I have taken some of the used characteristic toxic patterns that he identified and used them in the subheadings below. I have then expanded on his work to connect his patterns to those of toxic agers. Hopefully, these descriptions will be guidelines for baby boomers and successful future aging.

Starved for "Nurturance"

In a way it seems contradictory to say that the very people that chase others away with their hurtful words and body language are starved for nurturance, but they are. A self-centered focus leaves no room for self-love. Without self-love there is no love to give. Without love to give, little is received. Without nourishment, there is no such thing as successful aging.

Mistrusting and disbelieving in their own value, toxic agers perceive themselves as unworthy of receiving any positive strokes. Instead, negative strokes are unconsciously sought and substituted. The negative strokes are better than no strokes at all. At least with negative feedback, toxic agers get attention and feel alive. As in alcoholism, pain and anguished suffering are the norm, and the victim feels uncomfortable with success, praise, or love.

"Failuritis"

Living with constant, internal self-discounts for many years makes it difficult for toxic agers to practice self-nourishment. Rarely do they feel good internally. It is as if they "have a phobia about enjoying themselves" (1969, p. 4). By the time they are old, toxics are masters at rejecting compliments. Consistently, they find something wrong with themselves or how or what they did, preventing any positive input to help them feel better. It is like the older woman who won a quilting contest and when praised said, "If you had spent as many exhausting years working on quilts as I have, you'd win too."

"Explanationitis"

If you are ever around toxic agers for long, you will experience their incessant verbiage, endless details, and life history over and over as they try to explain themselves. Because their inner critic never ceases, they compulsively try to justify themselves and their actions, only to create more distance and stifle relationships.

Unable to Give

Another premise of Greenwald's is that toxics "seem incapable of making another person feel good. They are unable to give to others in a straightforward, honest fashion with no strings attached" (1968, p. 3). Any joy that another experiences from a toxic is usually short-lived or conditional, and if a toxic does do something for others, the situation is usually spoiled by generous complaining about all the effort and energy it took and what was wrong with it. The comments instead instill a sense of indebtedness and expected reciprocation.

Poor Receivers

Toxics have difficulty receiving. They seem unable to graciously accept a compliment, a gift, a service, or one's time or care without some distressing, passive-aggressive, guilt hooks. For example, those of you who have a toxic client or parent living in a skilled or congregate care facility know what it means when you make a concerted effort to visit regularly. Invariably, as you leave (especially if family), the comment is dropped in that familiar plaintive whiny tone, "I'm sure you could make the effort to visit more often if you really wanted to. But that's all right, I'll just sit here and be lonely."

Many toxic agers are physically self-reliant and live independently but will require help at times. Often, if this help comes from a service provider, they will gush with appreciation, but if offered by the adult child, there is nothing he or she can do that is "right." Adult children are often treated as though slaves, unable to walk away. Day and night, sometimes hourly, toxic agers will call a son or daughter to complain about some petty item or hysterically demand that he or she drop everything and come immediately. It's an emergency! Then, despite the fact that the commands are followed explicitly, only wailing is heard upon arrival. He or she did not get there fast enough. In addition, the call is no longer important (see case examples in chapter 5).

Preventing a stress crisis here is critical. Because situations like this are volatile, they can impede professional service or treatment. Consequently, it is advisable to work with the co-Victim, being constantly alert for signs and signals that enable the toxicity to continue.

Obligation Instillers

Practiced toxic agers of all cultures are masters at the self-sacrificing martyr game, controlling others by making them feel obligated and grateful. If service providers or adult children refuse a request, they are "made to feel guilty and selfish" (1968, p. 3). If they comply, and it is a game, they become co-Victims and accessories to the toxic behavior.

Greedy and Insatiable

Toxic agers "hunger for inner peace and contentment" (1968, p. 4) but are incapable of finding it. Their self-dissatisfaction accelerates a greed that may eventually take the form of a compulsion. It becomes an endless, insatiable reaching for an impossible goal. The more the toxics demand and push for their perceived illusion, the more they "fall into a state of depression, despair, and futility" (1968, p. 4). It is a cyclic, reinforcing, feedback loop that generates the negative energy often felt by those around them. As one daughter-in-law commented, "She's like a black cloud hanging over everything."

Insecure and Fearful

Much of the fear felt by toxic agers comes from any threat to their perceived safety and security. Always on guard, they are much less willing to take risks than the average person is. Instead of seeing change as something to stimulate their aliveness, as any successful ager would, they immediately respond with rapid, excessive, and inappropriate language and behavior, a response pattern that simply exposes their anxiety and fear. It also reveals the toxic's tendency to defensively overreact and to exhibit disowned hostility and submerged anger churning inside. It is as if toxics have to keep the lid on for fear they will explode, a feeling that can be terrifying for the toxic ager. If the professional and caregiver are not aware of this tendency and not prepared to protect themselves from the onslaught, they can easily perceive the attack as vehement and personal.

"Controlitis"

Horney calls it "rigid self-control" (1945/1992, p. 17). Greenwald calls it "control madness" (1968, p. 5). One of the greatest blocks to toxic agers' ability to nourish themselves is their unrealistic need to secure their environment before they can relax. Ordinary daily activities are joyless unless everything is "just so" and feels safe. With little frustration tolerance for anything that does not meet their standards, order, and expectations, toxic agers can attain a "chronic attitude of squeezing and inhibiting their spontaneity and naturalness . . . like a straightjacket" (Greenwald, 1969, p. 8).

Controlitis is also used by toxic agers as a way of holding themselves together. The fear of "losing it" incessantly infiltrates their daily thoughts. The straightjacket worn to contain this fear is more palatable if it is projected onto victims through a position of power. Seeing themselves in others and inflicting rigid unrealistic controls makes it possible for toxics to deny their own fears, as demonstrated so clearly by the toxic employee in chapter 5.

Even without power positions, toxic agers will maintain control through manipulation. An example is the way they seduce people into friendships and involvements. Once the persons are won over, relationships sink into situations totally dominated by the toxic person. In operation it is the Victim/Persecutor game (see chapter 10 for psychological games). Freedom and integrity are now sacrificed in order to maintain the game. The lament then follows, "Why do I allow her to do this to me?"

Emotional Constipation

Closely associated with controlitis are the toxic ager's inhibition and suppression patterns. Toxics must maintain an outer masklike tranquility in order to cover up emotional tensions inside that create a "chronic pressure which strains the whole organism" (Greenwald, 1969, p. 7). Although they appear strong, their insides are like inner volcanoes of withheld feelings ready to erupt. Over time, facial and body characteristics develop, such as hard, deep lines about the face, a jaw locked in tension, squinty eyes, and a loud high voice with rapid delivery. Eventually, the older skilled toxics are so effective in controlling their emotions that no expression will show. Internally, however, the pain and tension are still there, suppressed, never releasing the bearer from their torment.

Helpless Victim

Interestingly, it is the toxic agers who perceive themselves as helpless, powerless Victims in the typical control scenario. Their excessive need to feel safe is generally hidden and deceptively subtle. They pretend to be innocent victims, needing to be rescued by someone else. In such instances, unfortunately, the *Rescuer* ultimately becomes the Victim, and the destructive toxic game goes on and on—endlessly—as long as there is someone willing to play or until one of the players stops. (See Karpman's Triangle and game identification in chapter 10.)

"Maybe someday, mother will be capable of standing on her own two feet," is one daughter's wishful plea. That is not reality. Such avoidance thinking and projection only deepen the trap as the Rescuer daughter hooks in, again, to the co-Victim role and keeps the game going.

When you, as gerontology professionals, take on the responsibility of a toxic client, constantly watch for *signals* of psychological game playing in yourself. Games are unconscious, and you, as the helper, are just as vulnerable to the "bad feeling" aftereffects of the game as are the adult children. In addition, be constantly alert for the role switches. You too can be caught in the Victim role, with the toxic ager as the *Persecutor.*

Oppressive Nature and Attitude

The negative energy of toxics is unmistakable. It can permeate an entire room or environment like heavy, choking smoke. One can feel it the minute you enter a room. If positive energy is not upheld, the negative energy will consume whatever goodwill is present. Notice the next time a known and adept toxic ager is present. Watch how people are sucked into the toxic's games, in direct relation to the adroitness of the toxic and the vulnerability of the Victims. Toxic agers have had many years to fine-tune their toxicity skills. With this practice they have become masters at projecting their dark shadow side onto others. Observant and aware individuals, when subjected to such contamination, can see and feel the depressing seductiveness and misery-making nature of such an encounter. A malaise, such as John Steinbeck's, can be avoided. Just keep in mind that toxicity is contagious to the unaware, especially in the formative years of the young.

Ineffective Communicators

Not surprisingly, toxic agers do not listen. They do not express themselves appropriately and responsibly or with genuine feelings. To cover up these inabilities, it is common for toxics to maintain a flow of meaningless and incessant verbiage. Those on the receiving end listen politely for fear of offending them, but toxics are so absorbed in themselves, their conversations miss any quality of self-expression, giving, or hearing skills. Often, says Greenwald, there is a "close correlation between the meaninglessness of their conversation and the rapidity or quantity of words they disgorge" (1968, p. 5). Toxics simply cannot, or will not, connect honestly with others.

Prefer Being Miserable

One can easily get the impression that toxic agers like being miserable. For example, observe how secure and less anxious they are when those around them are frustrated and unhappy. To keep these negative strokes coming, advanced toxics tend to surround themselves with people who will reinforce their negative patterns and games. If asked directly, however, toxics will vehemently deny this penchant. Why? Because they are unaware of what they are doing. It has become an unconscious habit; it has the ease of the familiar. It is a known they can trust, not necessarily what they really want.

Greenwald adds that toxics "tend to experience increased anxiety, insecurity and frustration when they encounter happy, joyous people who are full of life. Their intense discomfort with self-nourishing, healthy personalities may become unbearable" (1968, p. 6). The only emotional payoff for habituated toxics seems to be either attempting to pull other persons down into their own state of misery or withdrawing from healthy people and getting comfort from their own kind. According to Horney, this is an achievable effort to do away with inner conflicts and to create an artificial harmony (1945/1992, pp. 16, 33).

Reflections

Yes, it was serendipitous that I impulsively picked up Karen Horney's book *Our Inner Conflicts*, especially when I realized she was 60 years of age when it was published. Now, as I turn 70, I am not only rediscovering some of the work of one of the most original psychoanalysts after Freud, but I am amazed at how closely her theories, and many of the descriptions of neurosis, resemble those of toxicity.

Fifty years ago, neurosis was the "in" word, especially after Horney's book *The Neurotic Personality of Our Time* (1937) hit the public market. The use of the word "neurosis" as a designated diagnostic term, however, has not been prevalent since DSM-II (APA, 1968). Nevertheless, its reappearance in the 1990s is an interesting connection with toxicity. The constant reruns of the cycles never cease to fascinate me as another example of how the young can learn from the old.

Toxicity occurs in relationships, stirred by what goes on inside. As Moody said, according to the basic insight of Buddhism, "It is our fear of experiencing ourselves directly and fully that creates for us the unnecessary suffering of human life. Neurosis, in fact, could be defined as unnecessary suffering" (1997, Spring, p. 1).

To go beyond this "unnecessary suffering," it depends on how much each of us chooses to awaken to the person we really are, embracing all of what is found inside (shadow, warts, conflicts, and all), accepting the accompanying vulnerability, and fully loving the whole Self, and others, unconditionally. A difficult task, but the task of old age. What a gift we can give the baby boomers if we, as older adults, show them we can do it.

Summary

Why the focus on toxic agers? With the demographics of our nation and the arrival of baby boomer agers, this anomaly of aging can no longer be ignored. Whether we like it or not, to some degree we each have the potential within us to become toxic. It is a personality development disturbance that can be prevented if we wake up to its neurotic tendencies, recognize the symptoms, understand the interplay of personality forces, and choose to nourish ourselves until we feel safe, secure, and loved enough to be able to change our inner thoughts, perceptions, and distorted self-image.

Horney's classic work (1937, 1945/1992) on personality disturbance and neurosis in the late 1930s and 1940s is found to be remarkably similar to descriptions of toxicity. Horney is convinced that disruptive inner personality conflicts can be resolved by changing the conditions within the personality that brought them about.

Greenwald, who initiated the early work on toxicity in the late 1960s, proclaims that self-nourishment is the way to bring about the change in the personality conditions described by Horney. Listed were 14 characteristics of toxicity proposed by Greenwald to aid you in the identification of symptoms and in teaching early intervention and prevention.

Personal shadow work, a concept of Jung's, is also a way to become alert to the inner personality conflicts and characteristics that plague the toxic ager and, if philosophically expanded, the nation (see chapter 8 regarding personality types and theories).

Facing the Options

With 75 million baby boomers turning 70 in 20 years, plus the expectation of an aging population containing large, multiethnic groups and cultures, a different aging dynamic must be realistically faced. Denial will not produce successful aging, nor will ignoring the toxic agers who can teach the younger generations much about the pain of living with inner turmoil and conflict. Alertness and attention must be given to the presenting signs and characteristics of toxicity, to transcending the idealized false ego self and finding our true selves, and to avoiding the displacement of our self-generating fears and their unconscious projections onto others that only create misery instead of harmony. We have a choice: a pattern of self-nourishment or a pattern of self-destruction and toxicity.

Chapter 3

How Do We Know They Are Toxic?

*The good that I would
I do not,
but the evil that I would not,
that I do*

—Romans 7:19

People ask, "How do I know if someone is toxic?" A flippant answer would be, "*You'll know.* If you have to ask, you haven't dealt with one."

Actually, there is no reliable assessment tool at this time. In fact, I am hoping there never will be an exact diagnostic instrument for toxicity because I firmly believe professional judgment and client interaction on a case-by-case basis is the most accurate.

Nevertheless, I'm well aware that a discussion starter accelerates movement in any case, so I'm offering two initial tools for your use as appropriate. These are rudimentary, so be creative, even develop your own.

First is a list of some signs of toxicity (p. 41) (gathered over years of experience, observation, processing, and research) that may provide some guidelines. Use it as a checklist, but remember, your own observations over time are still the most trustworthy. The second is a self-assessment toxicity indicator (p. 43) to help individuals determine their propensity toward toxicity if they are interested. Neither is perfected, or validated.

Behavioral Characteristics

Toxicity, like neurosis, can be found in varying degrees in all of us. A toxic person, as discussed in this book, manifests a persistent behavioral style that will consist of a majority of the indicators listed later. Although a possible character or personality type disorder, toxicity is not a medical disease and cannot be precisely measured as such. Instead, it is seen as an unhealthy personality, fixated at an early developmental stage, that has produced a dysfunctional, relational lifestyle. Because toxicity is developmental, its pattern of behavior can be prevented through early intervention, education, awareness, and personal commitment to change. Traditional psychotherapy that treats symptoms is usually ineffective.

Labeling of Toxic Agers

Quick and expedient labeling of toxicity can be a pitfall. I caution you against it. The purpose of the label is not to stereotype the older adults but to awaken you to the anomaly so you will know what to expect, how to handle it, how to avoid absorption of the toxin yourself, and how to let it serve as a strategy facilitator.

Your major responsibility is to understand toxic agers, not diagnose or cure them. In fact, there is no cure, only healing, and that occurs solely if toxics choose to heal themselves. Obviously, this creates a challenging role for you.

Professional Assessments

Toxic behavior is chronic and needs observation time. Among the many clues, look for a long-term pattern of self-misery and desperate need to control, Victim consciousness, a negative energy drain on those with whom your client interacts, and the family response to the behavior, especially the adult child co-Victim and likely coclient. Change may occur if the repetitive system of game interplay between co-Victims is stopped.

When making your assessment, notice your client's nonverbal signs and your own intuitive reaction. Paying attention to your inner sense is crucial. What is going on inside you and how you personally and professionally respond to the toxic's seductive game bait are paramount. Observe these closely.

Nonverbal Signs

Nonverbal signs were referred to earlier in another chapter but are specified here to emphasize their importance. The list of verbal signs may be long and oppressive, but the nonverbal signs of a toxic are more seductive and critical. Guilt-laden feelings are the product. The "feel sorry for me" looks, the glares, the scowls, the tightened jaw and fist, the turned back, the walking away, the withdrawal, the shut or locked door, the nonexistent hug or touch, the tone of voice, the pitch, the whining, the sad facial expression, the turned-down mouth, the piteous sighs, the incipient pauses, and those dreaded silences are typical. To the sensitive, the nonverbal message from the toxic penetrates. "It's a look," as one senior center director described it, "as if there is no life in there." Alertness is basic.

Assessment Checklist

Toxicity is acted out in generally increasing degrees of negative interactive behavior. Review the items below and check those applicable to your client. If more than half of the items are marked there is a chance toxicity is present. Firm results, however, must be confirmed by other assessments.

_____ Incessant complaining
_____ Projection of own negative self-characteristics onto others to avoid dealing with them
_____ Constant blaming of others for own personal problems. (It is always "_their_ fault.")
_____ Does not listen; unable or unwilling to really "hear" others or ourselves
_____ Excessively critical of others, especially of own children who never do anything "right"
_____ Defense mechanism expert; skillfully uses at least four of the following: denial, displacement, emotional insulation, help-rejecting complaining, isolation of affect, passive aggression, projective identification, rationalization, reaction formation, and repression (see Glossary). (Circle ones that match)
_____ Drains energy of those with whom they associate
_____ Starved for nourishment and love, yet nonreceptive to same
_____ Tormented by inner conflict between true self and idealized false self
_____ Dogmatic, domineering, and inflexible
_____ Arbitrarily knows what's right and says so
_____ Skillful negative manipulator
_____ Controlling, both subtle and overt
_____ Speaks inappropriately and loudly
_____ Pits family members against each other
_____ Self-centered, all attention focused on self; if ignored, a martyred withdrawal
_____ Demands instant compliance to wishes
_____ Claims no ownership or responsibility for behavior
_____ Constantly overreacts, often over small things
_____ Radiates a negative energy
_____ Endless explanations to justify actions
_____ Quick with the putdowns and discounts
_____ "Game" player; easily "hooks" or is "_hooked_" into psychological games

_____ Passive-aggressive responses
_____ Unable to be vulnerable with others or form lasting and
close relationships

Personal Signs

_____ Low self-esteem
_____ Feel and act victimized
_____ Unable to nurture self
_____ A depressive attitude
_____ Self-pitying
_____ Emotionally insecure
_____ Suspicious, may have signs of paranoia
_____ Close-minded and rigid
_____ Self-deceiving and deluding
_____ Compulsive and insatiable
_____ Suppresses feelings
_____ Not honest or direct in communications

Public Behavior Signs

_____ Charming to outsiders when wants to be; puts on "act"
in public
_____ May be a "pillar of the church" or community, even
volunteer
_____ Frequently interrupts or disturbs a meeting or conversation to control direction

Note. Again, when you use this checklist with clients, patients,
coworkers, friends, family, or yourself, do it with caution. It is
only a guide. It does not determine toxicity. Personal exposure,
experience, and listening to your own inner sense are still your
best assessment tools.

Some of the descriptions may have touched you personally by
describing someone you know, someone you love, someone you
are attempting to help or avoid, or possibly some of your own
shadow traits. That is natural. Just pay attention. Observe and get

in touch with your feelings. Understanding and discerning any unseen forces that may affect your professional or personal effectiveness is critical.

Depending on the degree of toxicity, some toxic agers can be helped, some cannot. Some are feared, all are difficult. The key is to know what you are dealing with, to maintain a professional nonattachment that balances caring and objectivity, and to refuse to play the toxic games.

How Would I Know If I Am Toxic?

Adult children exposed to the emotional abuse of toxicity when young are prime suspects for being toxic because it is passed down through the generations. Consequently, professionals who have, or had, toxic parents are automatically vulnerable and need to be doubly alert (as I was not) for possible countertransference. To deny your own toxicity; refuse to recognize or work through the symptomology; and allow yourself to get hooked into toxic games by neglecting constant self-observation, self-love, and self-nourishment are fuel for the contamination and deterioration of your own professional efforts.

To help you with this self-observation, I have devised an assessment tool that may aid you in determining your own toxic propensities if you suspect your background indicates it is appropriate. Remember, it is *not* a diagnostic instrument or the final word. It is merely a tool for you to gain personal insight and information to see if you are, to any degree, subject to some disowned toxic behavior.

Self-Assessment Toxicity Indicator

Note. This indicator is only a means to awaken self-insight. It is not a valid, or reliable, test. If you are honest with yourself, however, it will give you valuable information and stimulate new thinking. Use it as an exploration tool.

Scoring System

Because the scoring is strictly arbitrary, it is set up purely to give you some fun and to capture your inquiring spirit. Any validity is found only through what you give it. Score each statement on a scale of 1 to 5.

1 = Never, 2 = Rarely, 3 = Sometimes, 4 = Usually, 5 = Almost always

Add up the numbers to get your total score. Check the scoring key at the end for your results. (And, no peeking!)

_____ 1. Your family and others don't appreciate or value you.

_____ 2. You find you complain often over little things.

_____ 3. Few things seem to go right.

_____ 4. If it weren't for your childhood upbringing, you would be a happier person.

_____ 5. It is demeaning to accept help from others.

_____ 6. You resist an honest, direct confrontation in order to work through a conflict with others.

_____ 7. You wonder why you have so few friends.

_____ 8. You are suspicious of others' behavior toward you.

_____ 9. You feel safe and less anxious when you are in control of situations and your environment.

_____ 10. Misunderstandings are common with others.

_____ 11. You didn't feel your parents' love growing up.

_____ 12. You were abused verbally, emotionally, sexually, or physically as a child.

_____ 13. It would be so much easier if others would take responsibility for your decisions.

_____ 14. Growing up, you lived with a toxic adult.

_____ 15. Feelings were rarely allowed expression.

_____ 16. It is difficult for you to accept a compliment without an excuse or explanation.

_____ 17. If you do something for others, you hear yourself complaining about all the effort it took.

_____ 18. Few things meet your high standards.

_____ 19. You find yourself wishing for inner peace.

_____ 20. You are unable to express your needs to others.

_____ 21. You feel you have to make demands or push others into doing what you want.

_____ 22. Despite your intentions, you hear negative words coming out of your mouth before you realize it.

_____ 23. Inner turmoil, conflicts, and indecision are common.

_____ 24. Others say you overreact and become overly emotional. You don't understand what they mean.

_____ 25. You find it easy to get others to like you at first contact—if you want them to.

_____ 26. You feel you need to maintain control of your environment or surroundings in order to feel safe.

_____ 27. You find you have difficulty being really honest, open, and vulnerable with others.

_____ 28. You notice that you rarely compliment others, especially loved ones.

_____ 29. You feel more alive as the center of attention.

_____ 30. You observe that others feel you have criticized them when you only want things to be "right."

_____ 31. When you walk into a room, you automatically see what's wrong.

_____ 32. You have trouble nurturing yourself.

_____ 33. You feel uncomfortable around joyful people who continually see the bright side of life.

_____ 34. An inner voice is constantly telling you what you should do, should not do, or should not have done.

_____ 35. When something goes wrong, you instantly see what the other person did to cause it.

_____ 36. You have no idea what your personal needs are.

_____ 37. It is easy for you to find, and point out, the errors and mistakes others make.

_____ 38. You find it difficult to love the parts of yourself you can't tolerate and won't accept.

_____ 39. It's distressing not to be able to have fun like others.

_____ 40. When things aren't going your way, you get frustrated and either attract attention to yourself or deliberately withdraw.

_____ 41. As the years go by you find it increasingly more difficult to get others to meet your needs.

_____ 42. There are times when you feel so tense inside it's as
if you are going to explode. Therefore, you have to
maintain rigid control just to hold yourself together.
It's a constant fear.

_____ 43. As you get older, people seem more distant. It gets
very lonely.

_____ 44. Life is becoming more and more of a burden because
no one seems to appreciate or value you.

Remember. This is not a test. Its purpose is to stimulate awareness
and awaken you to personal tendencies that may be unconsciously
buried (a form of shadow work). If brought to light, these parts
may enhance your professional effectiveness plus enable you to
have more meaningful experiences with clients, parents, and life.

Scoring

Count up your total points. Now locate your classification. Be
sure to doublecheck your addition and then verify your score.
You intuitively know what is accurate, and you do not have to
agree with the results. Just use the classifications to further explore
what you learned from the exercise.

Classifications

0–44	Free
45–90	Immune
91–135	Exposed
136–180	Coming Down with
181–220	Full-Blown Case

Interpretations

Free	Terrific! No victimization in you
Immune	Great! Immunity reigns
Exposed	Hang in, prevention will prevail
Coming Down with	Still hope. Develop those coping skills
Full Blown Case	Hey! It's not over yet. Learn to love you

Cautions

If you scored in the first two classifications, don't be too smug. I'm sure there's a self-satisfied feeling despite the fact that this is not a diagnostic tool. Just having a means for assessment can in itself become a toxic tool if you use it to label either yourself or your clients. If the implications of the results are not processed, discussed, and used as a learning opportunity, little growth occurs. Make the statements help you understand yourself, or clients, and the hidden pain and angst uncovered, not just to diagnose.

If you scored in the middle classification, you are likely a child of a toxic, and a recovering one at that, who has worked through much of your own "stuff." Congrats! Just remember, it means a lifelong practice of vigilance and being on guard.

If you scored in the last two classifications, you will have a sense of what your clients (both the toxic ager and the adult child) are experiencing. You will know their pain and inner turmoil and how easy it is to deny and project it onto others. Process and explore your feelings, bring them to the light. Dealing with them honestly, in addition to nurturing and loving yourself (see chapters 13 and 14), will only make you a better professional. Once you have worked through your own defenses, you will be able to understand and manage the denial, the projections, and the rationalizations that naturally occur in yourself and in these clients. Plus, you'll be able to understand, and perhaps empathize with, the co-Victim relationship between a toxic parent and his or her adult child.

Summary

In essence, chapter 3 is a means for identifying toxicity in individuals. It provides some clues and two assessment tools: a checklist and a self-report indicator. They are offered to help you, as a professional in the gerontology field, discern possible symptoms of toxicity in your clients, or in yourself. Nonverbal, verbal, and personal and public behavioral signs are also described to enable a clearer appraisal.

Caution is given against quick labeling and diagnosing because the assessment tools have not been validated, nor are they reliable scientific measurements. Toxicity in agers is a new concept, and much needs to be learned. Your most reliable assessment is still your own experience, training, and intuition.

Chapter 4

Are Toxic Agers Found in All Groups?

Yes, older adults that behave as if they are toxic are found in every group and culture. These toxic agers are perceived as difficult and troublesome and in conflict with cultural norms and expectations. Humanity is known to possess a full range of personalities, behavior, and attitudes, both negative and positive. Older adults who live long enough can show their dark side when controls are lifted. Nevertheless, some groups will deny any negative aspects of aging: a form of positive ageism according to Palmore (1990). It all depends on whether the perceived behavior is accepted in the cultural environment of the older adult.

To research these groups, 14 minority psychotherapists, social workers, community and senior center directors, caseworkers, and other service providers were contacted or interviewed, or both. Those individuals gave hours of their time to help us begin to understand multicultural ethnic differences and perceptions.

Older adult minority group representatives were Latino (Mexican, Hispanic, and Cuban), Vietnamese, Native American, and Jewish. African Americans were not excluded. Their dispersement and small percentage (1%) of the demographics in the geographic area considered did not lend itself to representative research. Instead, I found several seasoned African American professionals directing large multiethnic community and senior centers. They were extremely helpful in recounting their experiences and observations with toxic agers.

Interview findings revealed some variations among the different older, minority adult groups, but more striking were the similarities. Recognition of toxicity in the agers did, however, vary depending on the role, training, and experience of the interviewees.

Psychotherapists

As with the White majority group, the psychotherapists interviewed in clinics serving minority groups said they saw very few elderly patients. Those they did see were usually involuntarily brought in during a state of crisis in which medication and hospitalization became the primary focus. No time could be spent on personality anomalies other than to note behavioral patterns to the family and refer out.

According to one Latino clinical director, "Problems are exacerbated because Latinos have a pattern of not bringing mental health issues to an agency. This makes treatment more difficult."

Community Centers

Services provided in community centers generally consist of meeting emergencies, finding housing and jobs, serving hot meals, and distributing government commodities, household items, and clothes. There is usually no staff for special programs for special age groups.

With the onset of the Welfare Reform Act in 1997, however, directors interviewed said they suddenly had an influx of seniors coming for food and services because they feared they would be losing federal benefits.

Yes, toxic elders were among their new recipients.

How did they handle them without special staff?

One director whose agency serves mostly Hispanics stated it succinctly:

> Because toxic agers are very demanding, loud, and complaining, our goal is to get them in and out as fast as possible. We tell them to sit down, to come on days when we are not so busy, and then assign a volunteer to sit with them outside under the trees, if possible, in order to ease their fears, talk with and listen to them, and help them feel comfortable.

Senior Centers

Services are the same in senior centers as they are in community centers except senior centers exclusively serve older adults age 60 and up and offer additional programs, classes, activities, and assistance, such as in-home care referrals, shared housing, and transportation designed specifically for the senior's special needs.

Participation in each senior center usually reflects the ethnic populations surrounding the center's location. An exception, however, is the Title III meal program that may at times serve a higher percentage of minorities than are proportionately found in the general population.

Nonetheless, according to the directors of these centers, ethnic elders have the reputation of not seeking support, asking for help, or participating in any groups in which their personal concerns are displayed. Examples of toxic agers, however, are still found among the members.

Multiethnic Senior Center

One director of a senior center located in an inner city with a high Hispanic ratio related accounts of two situations: a toxic participant and a toxic employee.

The first example was an 83-year-old male who migrated from Cuba. He served in the Marine Corps, "loved America," was gifted in music and singing, had a health problem, and practiced "schmoozing the higher ups." He was known for making the rounds of all the senior centers but constantly complained about all of their services and pitted them against each other. He demanded to be the center of attention, in a negative or positive sense; was controlling; and often initiated power struggles. He was called "a mean spirit."

An example of one of his power struggles occurred one day at lunch when the older man demanded that the director of the center move the flag in the next room so the man could see it from where he was sitting. Noting that the man was sitting at the only table from which he could not see the flag, the director asked the elder to chose a different place to sit. In a loud outburst, the toxic accused the director of having no respect for the flag and being unpatriotic. This immediately inflamed the other members, whereupon the director, who was a tall, large man, stood over the toxic and said firmly, "It isn't fair to the others to give you special treatment. You will abide by the rules like everyone else." The toxic finally did.

Another example is the case of a 68-year-old female, Hispanic staff person who had been employed at the center for 6 years before the director was hired. For 18 months he tried to work with her. Finally, he realized she was incapable of changing, would not listen, refused his suggestions and advice, lied about the finances, and was unfair in her treatment of members.

She worked at the center, 20 hours a week and one of her duties was the management of the government food-distribution program. As the staff person in charge, she maintained rigid control and order by acting like a "prison warden," walking around carrying her clipboard and key ring in an authoritative manner. Yelling out numbers was her system of dispensing food. The atmosphere was always frenzied because the seniors attempted to get the early numbers so they could obtain the "goodies" before she gave them to her "buddies."

One very blustery winter day the director arrived at the center to find a line of seniors who had been standing out in the cold for an hour and a half in order to be among the first to get the better food products. According to the toxic's rules, they could not come in until it was time to open the door.

The last straw was provided later by two situations. First, a blind man was sent away without food because he was not a senior and came on a day not scheduled for him to receive bread. Second, another man, whom the director had sent to her to receive food, was refused in an accusatory, abrasive, and hostile voice. "You've been here before!"

The staff person was fired, but not before she angrily complained to the director's boss. In outside meetings, she charged that the director was deliberately out to get her.

The above example of late-stage toxicity is typical. According to reports, this particular employee had changed when her husband died 17 years before. Bitter and feeling deserted and alone, she never forgave him for leaving her.

Hispanic Senior Center

In this small senior center, services to the Hispanic older adults were typical. When inquiries about toxicity were made, however, especially regarding emotional problems, the response was different.

"In our culture, you don't take on mother or father," proclaimed the female, Hispanic director. Adult children resist taking charge, and traditional therapy and group counseling is out of the question. Older parents, particularly toxics, face their deeper issues only when their body gives way. Their self-treatment is total denial, helped by alcohol and prescription drugs such as Valium (diazepam) and painkillers.

Americanized Hispanic adult children are often discouraged when confronted with toxic situations among their older adults, but if they are creative and can collaborate with a doctor, a priest, or another authority figure, the older Hispanics will usually listen.

Another perception of the Latino client was expressed by a Hispanic student-intern working for a countywide older adult mental health service. He agreed that Mexican Americans in general do not access mental health services and added that since Proposition 209 was approved in California, they were even less likely to seek help or go to senior centers for "fear of losing access to health care benefits."

He further added that with acculturation, there is a growing change in attitudes among the Hispanic, leading to fewer extended families. The same frustrations of the "Anglo sandwich generation" are now showing up, and, with the difficult ager especially, it is creating internal problems relative to family needs and dynamics.

Vietnamese Senior Center

According to the manager of a large, active Vietnamese senior center, toxic Asians "definitely exist."

Two things have intensified the presence of toxicity in Vietnamese elders: (1) cultural conflicts between the Vietnam-born elders and the American-born adult children and (2) the elders' loss of power and control.

In Vietnam, Confucian teachings are dominant. Elders are revered. No one is allowed to criticize them. Any other option or expectation other than to bow your head and accept the elders' demands is unthinkable.

The conflicts that arose when the second generation became Americanized were predictable. Those previously in power in Vietnam, such as one military general at the center, are insulted and offended if people don't listen and don't act when they speak. Once considered the bravest, wisest, and best loved, these older Asians now have to depend on their families and feel demeaned, resentful, and powerless. Their demands continue, but the children rebel. Relationships are strained. Nagging parents are no longer tolerated. Their previously stabilized roles are gone.

"After all I've sacrificed for you, how could you treat me this way?" are the endless wails.

Many of these parents are now using their Supplemental Security Income (SSI) money to move in with other older Vietnamese in order to share rooms and customs and live near a Buddhist temple where their opinion can be heard and respected, and they can "purchase" peace and advice from the revered priests.

Other toxic parents are financially subsidized and placed in residential care facilities by their children but then avoided and refused emotional support if the children feel they are being abused.

Nevertheless, that common guilt felt by most adult children of toxic parents is also seen in the Vietnamese community, as illustrated by the following example. This is the case of a woman in her mid-80's who was put in a nursing home by her four successful, all-Americanized professional children. After the placement, none of them went to visit, but "when the mother died, the children gave her a big, showy funeral."

To ease the cultural conflicts, special classes have been set up at the Vietnamese center to help both the elders and their children to understand each other and the divisive clashes. Still, toxicity is different. It does not seem to be exclusive to any culture. When elders make life difficult for their children, even a 70-year-old Vietnamese only son will resent it. In this case, the son got tired of his 99-year-old mother calling in the middle of the night from her nursing home demanding that he come over immediately to scratch her back because she had an itch.

Native American Center, Senior Program

Another conflict of values between cultures regarding elders is found with Native Americans. According to the director of the senior program, "respect for elders is bottom-line."

In the Native American culture, members have been taught that elders are to be treated with dignity, regardless of what happens. "No one is to yell at them, criticize them, or be firm with them. You must allow them to be whatever they are," continued the director. "Elders deserve to be any way they want. A younger person's role is to learn from them. They are our teachers."

When running a program, however, this value can create havoc if a toxic is involved and a "snowball effect" erupts in the group. An example was a recent bingo game.

It was the second time an elderly White toxic had come to the center to play bingo. Shortly after the game started, she began to yell and complain every time something was not the way she wanted it. Soon it became contagious. Others also started to complain. Halfway through the activities, the woman suddenly stood up and shouted, "These are piddly assed gifts. Why even bother to come here for them!"

By now, her outbursts had disrupted the entire hall. It was chaos. The caller, a young Native American, was simply adhering to his culture. For an hour and a half, he had simply "let the woman do her thing." Now, stunned by the consequences, the young man was at a loss. He had no idea what to do. Finally, he called in the program director.

Admitting it was "tough to do," the director, a Native American social worker, took the woman by the arm, led her outside, and firmly and directly told her such behavior was not tolerated. She would have to leave.

This was a moment of testing between two values. The director felt she had only one option. Her professional responsibility was the stability and peace of the center. It took precedence over cultural beliefs. In her social work training and experiences, the director had learned a different set of priorities and values.

Jewish Senior Center

There are four possible reasons why the director of the Jewish center first responded to my question regarding toxic agers with "Oh, we don't have any toxics. We have a wonderful group. It's close knit, we've been together for a long time, have a sense of belonging, and support each other." Then there was a pause. "Oh, maybe we have one or two isolated cases, but nothing serious. They don't become a public problem." Therein ended the inquiry.

The long-time social worker for the same program, however, had a different perception and experience. Considering the number of adult children she frequently counseled—helping them to assuage guilt and dysfunctional relational problems with their aged parents—she assured me toxic agers did exist in the group.

There were four possibilities for the two different perceptions and subsequent responses:

1. Intimacy of a close-knit group, and the loving, supportive attention given them, may give an extraverted toxic's ego exactly what it unconsciously needs, thereby discouraging any excessive acting out at the center.
2. Toxicity can be hidden from service providers and others who block out the dark side, don't want to see the negative

and thus perceive everything as rosy, and work hard to please their clients by giving them what they want.

3. The center director may have been protecting her image of the center, unconsciously resisting the release of anything she perceived as negative to the public.
4. Toxics are known for behaving differently in public if it is to their benefit.

Regardless, the different reactions support the initial hypothesis stated in the Preface: "People respond to others and things according to the way they perceive them" (Davenport, 1991, p. 6).

Summary

It can be assumed that toxic agers are found in all groups but only called toxic if the word is picked up and attached to the perception. In all humans, there is a light side and a dark side, and if positive ageism is not rampant, the dark toxic side will be recognized, sometimes tolerated, sometimes not.

Cursory research on the presence of toxicity in active, older adult, ethnic and religious minority groups, and how it is handled, was conducted through interviews with minority service providers, primarily in psychotherapy, community centers, and senior centers in Southern California. Groups examined were Latino, Hispanic, Vietnamese, Native American, and Jewish.

Some variations in the groups were discovered, but the similarities among the diversity were surprising.

For instance, regardless of ethnic and cultural or religious beliefs, most older adults (especially toxics) avoid psychotherapists; fear mental illness; refuse to share personal feelings and issues (in essence their dirty linen); deny emotional symptoms unless forced by illness, children, or some outside authority to face them; and defensively project their denials onto others.

In addition, the generational conflicts of immigrants and refugees—between the old country and the new, the old ways and the new—are universal. Children adapt, but the stress, fears, and loss of self-identity, control, esteem, and power roles among some of the elderly unleash hidden toxic tendencies. These children usually do not understand why their parents cling to old stability and safety and that their feelings of being unnecessary, unwanted, unloved, and unproductive are all triggers for toxicity.

The elderly in the groups examined seemed to feel rejected if adult children did not appreciate all the sacrifices made for them. In the toxic agers, this feeling swelled to martyrdom. Like their children, these elderly perceived themselves as emotionally abused. Miscommunication and trouble arose when they were unable to identify what they were feeling or know how to express it. Instead, it came out in the middle of the night in senseless phone calls to "scratch my back."

Self-concepts among the toxic agers also seem to uniformly degenerate into the negative energy of Victim consciousness. These agers perceive themselves as true victims. They respond as *Victims* (see the discussion on transactional analysis and the Karpman game triangle in chapter 10). Fear unconsciously drives toxic agers to frenetic and rigid control needs, desperately hanging on to the little personal power they perceive they have left.

Part II

Who Is Affected by Toxic Agers, and How?

You have to begin by liking yourself, and you have to like others more. If you don't have that feeling of living in an affectionate universe, I think you'll perish, simply out of bile and bitterness.

—Stanley Kunitz, age 87

Chapter 5

Impact on Professionals

New and seasoned service providers in a variety of programs in the gerontology field were interviewed in an effort to discover the kind of impact "old" and "old-old" toxic agers had on these professionals, their ability to deliver services, and their agencies. These professionals were directors of area agencies and senior centers; those with a master's degree in social work (MSWs) and licensed clinical social workers (LCSWs) in protective services, resource centers, and private practice; mental health therapists and marriage and family counselors (MFCCs); case managers in private and county mental health and social programs; public guardians; specialists in geropsychiatric units, adult day care, elder abuse, adult activity programs, ombudsman services, hospices, senior information and referral services, and family in-home care; college professors and counselors; and practitioners in home health care, home meal drivers, and community aides. Some services were state and federally mandated, some were nonprofit, and some were private.

All 48 contacts and interviewees were asked if they had toxic agers in their programs and, if so, to describe the toxic behavior and its impact. All but the elder law lawyers, the representative of one senior center, and one public health educator acknowledged that they worked directly with toxic agers. The sample also revealed that seven (15%) of the service providers interviewed were daughters of toxic mothers and one was the divorced spouse of a toxic alcoholic. This number seemed relatively high compared with my estimate that 4 or 5% of the current aging population was toxic.

Where Are Toxics Found?

Almost universally, toxic agers are found in all areas where older adults receive direct services. An exception is with indirect services. For example, in elder law the contacts are primarily with the adult child seeking power of attorney, and the attendant conservatorship paperwork, not with the toxic ager.

The same exception can be found in public education programs or at the college or university level, where the older adults themselves help organize, manage, and implement the activities. Examples are continuing education programs geared to stimulate mental and social development and wellness. When asked about toxic agers, the response was, "We probably have some, but they aren't comfortable here for very long, and generally leave." The upbeat attitudes and *productive* energy at this type of challenging program leave little room for the negativity and Victim consciousness of toxic agers.

General Feedback

Although there seemed to be a persistent core pattern for toxic behavior among the aged, the impact on the professionals varied, depending on the number of years of exposure to toxics, their perception of toxic behavior, their own self-confidence and freedom in being able to develop creative coping skills, the number of toxic agers in their caseloads, and whether they themselves were children of a toxic parent.

Facing Reality

None of the professionals interviewed had specific training in dealing with toxic agers. It was not required in their job descriptions, nor was it available. Without training, most were forced to work out their own solutions. When pushed to the limit and faced with lengthy complaining phone calls, loud outbursts, and interruptions; constant fault finding, whining, and sniping; and other behavior that disrupted their efforts, they often found themselves discouraged and distressed and their energy consumed.

For many, working with the toxic agers seemed nonproductive. Survival and expediency became the goals. The result was negative coping. Toxics were avoided, circumvented, blocked, or (if possible) referred to someone else. Practicality often superseded desired service. If the toxicity was in an advanced state, the caseload excessive and intense, the staff support inadequate, and the primary focus crisis intervention, dealing with toxic agers was simply too time consuming and cost ineffective to attempt to do more than contain the problems. Long-term, sustainable results were no longer an option. The focus became only that which was attainable.

Typical Professional Responses to Toxic Agers

The more I listened to the professionals' and service providers' choice of words to describe their encounters with toxic agers, the more intently I felt their sense of helplessness. With rapid-fire feedback, the words would flow: frustrating, disruptive, spoiled, manipulative, chase people away, don't cooperate, self-centered, demanding, time consuming, constantly complaining and blaming others, paranoid, closed to change, must be a chemical imbalance in their brains, rehash the same thing over and over, never learned to let go, passive-aggressive, selfish, dependent, and unwilling to help themselves.

Just questioning these service providers about toxic agers seemed to stir unforgettable experiences. Descriptive phrases continued to pour out, as if in a cathartic release after finding someone who finally understood. Commonly heard were the following: They have learned over the years that this behavior is the way to get what they want; alienate everyone; want all the attention; see themselves as always right; want what they want NOW; feel so abused they don't see what they are doing to themselves and others; don't perceive themselves as being the cause of the problems; take their unhappiness out on others; are dysfunctional and unrealistic in resolving issues; do not *adapt*; are always negative; have a fighter personality; and are irritating and challenging.

As Steinbeck would say, they are "sad souls!"

Impact Examples

By now, as a service provider reading this, I suspect your reactions vary from relief in knowing you are not alone in your feelings to a fear of what you are getting into. If you are new in the gerontology field and have had no training in this area, strive to perceive working with toxic agers as a new challenge and adventure from which you can continue to grow professionally.

The following case examples will give you some insight and exposure to actual situations, plus some knowledge of what to expect. The hope is that this might help you understand the frustration, anxiety, guilt, and possible anger you may feel when attempting to serve toxics.

Organization of Cases. To facilitate easier reference points, case examples are identified by specifically listed categories, such as new caseworkers, senior centers, public services, private practice, special services, multiple issues (differential diagnoses), caregiver support services, and residential and retirement communities.

New Caseworkers

Professionals new on the job will find experiences with toxic agers vary. Nevertheless, each situation will be a learning opportunity, even though at the time it may not be perceived as such.

For example, one situation I heard of was a community worker who had only been on the job for a few weeks. In tears she quit, crying, "These people are driving me crazy."

Inquiring as to the circumstances, I was told, "She's young and doesn't have the tolerance and patience to deal with these bitchy types."

True, she may not have had the tolerance and patience, or even be right for the profession, but she did have the right to be appropriately trained for the task.

Labeling Helped. The second situation had a happier ending. It was 1989 when I put the label "toxic" on the difficult agers I had been interviewing for my dissertation, but it was several years later, after a presentation I made at a professional meeting on toxic agers, that a young social worker came up to me with an indescribable look of relief on her face. Her eyes shone as she confessed,

> I was really beginning to think there was something wrong with me! Until this morning I was afraid I would have to get out of the gerontology profession. You see, there were a couple of elderly people I just couldn't deal with. In fact, I've been ashamed because I've been avoiding them for weeks, and my boss is beginning to put the pressure on. Now that I know what toxic behavior is and can put a label on it, I know what to expect and how to deal with it.

Then, with a smile and an anxiety releasing sigh she said, "And it sure helps to know the problem isn't me. Thanks!"

I could have hugged her. She gave validation to my perception that identifying toxicity in agers helps everyone involved: the service providers, the adult children, and the elders themselves. If you know what you are dealing with, you can learn how to manage your response to it.

Yet, to step out and label anything negative about older adults seemed risky at the time, despite the fact toxicity has little to do with normal aging. There is always the chance that labeling can be taken as a prejudicial putdown instead of a tool intended to help us recognize and acknowledge that there is a disowned, undeveloped, and unacknowledged part in all of us, a shadow side that eventually breaks through, to some degree or another, when usual controls are weakened. It is a label that will hopefully jolt us, as professionals, to shift our perception on how to serve, and love, those who appear unlovable.

Senior Centers

Interestingly, to the seasoned service providers (particularly the long-term directors of senior centers), the word "toxic" brought forth quite a different response from that of new workers. To the directors, the word stimulated an "ah yes" knowing look and sigh. They did not have to be told the symptoms; they knew immediately to what I was referring, and to whom, although they did not call them toxic. Instead it was, "Oh, you mean _____ !"

Often during the interviews, the directors gave specific descriptions of the toxic behavior, and from their tone of voice and facial expressions, it was clear the presence of these emotional abusers was troublesome. Having them in a congregate or group setting was definitely not the preferred choice. At best it was disruptive, at worst, devastating.

Veteran directors recalled the early days of the 1970s, when both they and the senior center concept were new. Not expecting, or knowing how, to manage toxicity at the time, the unruly, disturbing behavior and negative attitudes of these agers often contaminated the whole program and restricted them from attending any group activities.

The directors also said that they appreciated being able to give the behavior a name because they felt it would make it easier to recognize the symptoms and know how to work with them. It meant others might be able to avoid the trial-and-error struggles and stress they experienced in those early days trying to cope with these individuals. It also meant treatment, not survival, might be the prime motivator. Nevertheless, because of their effort, practical strategies were created by these directors over time and are described in Part IV.

Many of these directors admitted, however, that even after 20 to 25 years, if they let down their guard or were tired, the toxic agers could still "get to them." Then the days became long and hard. If they could identify the toxic symptoms early, however, they were able to redirect, control, or remove the behavior for the sake of the others, as well as condition themselves against feeling personally attacked.

To you directors, we are grateful. Much can be learned from your dedicated persistent efforts and determination. You became a reservoir of information, tolerance, and understanding regarding the variables and differences so representative of all active elders. You, in a sense, have commissioned other readers to remember that each older person, especially the toxic, needs to be accepted and treated like the unique individual he or she is.

Public Services

Area Agency on Aging

Found in all states, Area Agency on Aging (AAA) offices and programs are mandated by the Federal Older Americans Act to be responsible for the development of comprehensive and coordinated systems of service for those age 60 and over. Organization and delivery of services vary in each location according to population size and need. All, however, are required to monitor distribution of funds and contract out services, as well as serve as the leader, chief advocate, and focal point for aging services in general.

Even the directors of these large agencies feel the impact of toxic agers. When asked about personal interactions with these individuals, one director smiled and said,

> Oh yes! There's one that disrupts every meeting. She calls the office frequently, but I have my secretary handle that. Actually, it's tougher on her. If the toxic ager approaches me, I just put the palm of my hand out toward her, shake my head, and walk away.

Again a piece of evidence that toxic agers affect all levels of gerontology service, each person creatively responding in whatever way works best for them.

Another function of AAA and some local programs is to provide or contract for the provision of services that enable frail seniors to remain independent and in their homes. These services include home meals, transportation to medical appointments, in-home support services, and case management. Volunteers deliver the home meals; case managers are assigned to assess the needs of, write a care plan for, and follow up on at-risk clients.

The whining, complaining, and blaming tendencies of toxic agers are common experiences for these community-based, long-term-care workers. Eventually, most adapt and some learn to cope, but they all say, "You never get used to it."

Difficulties usually arise when these caseworkers are not trained to manage the complicated, troublesome cases they feel compelled to serve. Such cases are commonly long term and complex. They are the ones other agencies discharge after learning, the hard way, that they are unable to help. The negative attitudes, resistance, and noncompliant behavior of the toxics make attempts to serve ineffective and unrewarding.

As one home care nurse reported (the only worker who could manage this particular toxic client),

> I get paid $24 an hour to sit for 40 minutes once a month to listen to this woman rant, rave, and complain. Then I help her as best I can and leave. I see to it she gets home meals and transportation to the doctor. That's all I can do.

Most agencies have a right to refuse services to a noncompliant client, but, feeling obligated, caring, and challenged, a new agency or worker will sometimes unwittingly take on a discharged case in a determined effort to be helpful. Unfortunately, it is only a matter of time before they too feel frustrated, inadequate, and distressed. Toxics can be unswervingly enticing during an initial contact, luring those who tend to Rescue into their toxic games (see chapter 10). The trap is set, workers unconsciously become co-Victims, and the game continues, only the players have changed. Big "R" Rescuing (see Karpman's Triangle in chapter 10) is a pitfall for almost every overly caring new worker.

Psychologically, toxic clients cannot be helped. They will change only if and when they choose to do so. That choice, however, rarely occurs before they no longer can find someone who is willing to play their toxic games. That someone must be immune to the game hooks and willing to interrupt the *toxic loop*.

Advanced toxics usually have multiple problems and are masters at exhausting helpers and resources. Each new worker or agency understandably succumbs to a toxic client's presented problems initially, only to eventually feel inept, defeated, and exhausted. In addition to drained energy, these workers often experience frustrations that are immediately projected onto the releasing or referral agency, subsequently creating undefined and negative professional relationships (an example of unconscious countertransference and toxic contamination).

Another factor to be considered is the hidden costs of attempting to provide care to unresponsive clients, costs that go undetected by providers and managed care policymakers.

Older Adult Protective Services

State laws mandate the reporting of abuse throughout the nation; however, services may vary from state to state. Because no statistical data under the term "toxic" are available, no specific numbers regarding toxic agers are quotable. Based on many years of experience, however, the director of one agency ventured to guess that emotionally abusive agers constitute about 10% to 15% of the caseload, again much higher than that 4% to 5% I speculated would be found in the normal older population.

Several theories exist as to the cause of the high incidence of elder abuse by children. Some believe it is a learned experience and "payback time," a sort of retribution for the past. Because abuse is an experienced part of the life history of toxic families, it could be expected that a toxic ager, living in a family already stressed to its limit, would have an aggravating impact on a care-providing relationship. I sense it also goes even deeper. To me, the abuser and abusee become co-Victims. They are enmeshed. Neither is capable of nourishing or loving himself or herself (or each other). Therefore, they unconsciously take their fears, anger, and distress out on each other, each in his or her own way.

As one director added, "The parent comes in as a nice old man, and then the son says, 'Oh yeah! He's been a bastard all my life.'"

A major purpose of the Older Adult Protective Services (APS) is to serve and protect the elder person in the home, as well as pick up the pieces if the adult child caregiver should leave. Understood in this is the fact that no law says the child *must* take care of the parent. To walk away, however, is too difficult a choice for most children, despite the degree of toxicity. Consequently, stress and burnout are common. If the adult child should choose to take on the responsibility of parental care, such as power of attorney or guardianship, however, it becomes a legal issue and the circumstances change.

If APS is called in, the agency's first responsibility is to assess the situation, work with the police and the civil attorneys, and refer out to supportive services. Secondary is the psychosocial need. Here some work can be done with long-term cases, but APS is required to have multiple reports before they can become intrusive with a family. At the onset of a case, APS cannot go beyond the ager's behavior or be involved in any family dynamics. Crisis intervention is the primary focus.

It is the toxic ager's behavior, however, that compounds the difficulties APS professionals already face in making complicated differential assessments. These assessments include alcoholism, depression, dementia, the effects of multiple and undeclared medications, and malnutrition, plus physical and emotional abuse, neglect, and exploitation.

Considering growing caseloads, the demanding, argumentative, and noncompliant behavior of toxic agers self-limits the full use of the protection system. It is as if these emotional abusers intend to be difficult and make it almost impossible for the social workers to serve them. Nonetheless, APS must stand on the side of the elder at all times. The adult child must either learn to cope or assume the consequences of a choice to continue the care of the parent.

Public Guardian's Office

An investigative arm of the courts, the Public Guardian's Office is an agency of last resort. The judicial system's preference is to find a family member or friend "willing and able" to act as a conservator, not to have the government take on the responsibility. According to one deputy public guardian, finding a friend for two thirds of the older adults referred, mostly for dementia, is possible. Of the remaining one third referred, however, investigative deputies estimate that almost one third of these older adults would also fall into the category of toxic agers. Again, an excessive percentage of toxics.

> One example is an 82-year-old widowed female whose children reported that they had tried to help their mother for years. According to the case report, the mother rarely, if ever, accepted the children's help with medical care, payment of bills, home maintenance, shopping, transportation, or money management. Instead, the mother complained that the children never helped her, accused them of trying to take advantage of her, and was critical of everything they tried to do. When a need for conservatorship arrived, the children had had it. They proclaimed they were no longer willing, even with court authority, to be responsible for their mother. They had tried everything they knew. The relationship was severed.

Private Practice

Individual Counseling

One-on-one work of any depth with toxic agers depends inevitably on the personality, training, personal confidence, self-trust, compassion, and spirituality of the professional involved, as well as the toxic ager's willingness to work. Toxics often, like children, intuitively "see right through" an authority figure, then zero in immediately on his or her weak spot. They are noted for their ability to push buttons and to talk incessantly without listening or seeming to take a breath. As implied earlier, toxics resist and vehemently reject any visible, or direct, therapeutic help. Well-honed defense mechanisms often negate any probable progress professionals may hope to attain.

From my experience, especially with advanced toxicity, individual counseling can be ineffective and time consuming. If the therapist happens to be a son or daughter of a toxic aged parent, psychotherapy becomes almost useless unless the therapist has worked through his or her own toxicity, a difficult challenge at best.

Therapist As an Adult Child of a Toxic Parent

The previous observation was reinforced by one MFCC, a daughter of a toxic mother, and two therapist friends who also were daughters of toxic mothers. The first friend was so entangled with her mother she couldn't protect herself and was off work for a month. It was not until her mother died that the daughter was released from the toxic game loop.

The other therapist was still desperately striving to deal with her situation and be effective, but to no avail. She accomplished only the depletion of her own energy.

The interviewee herself stated that she worked through most of her toxic entrapment in graduate school after attempting to assist a patient who tried to transfer her toxic anger and guilt to the then student counselor. Unaware of what was happening and not being able to put her own frustrations and anger aside, the sessions ended only when the patient overdosed on painkillers. Looking back, the MFCC said she tried so hard to work with this woman, then realized finally that, at the time, she did not have the awareness, strength, or understanding to face her own involvement and countertransference complications.

Special Social Services

It is apparent that there are a number of special services available in today's society for the older adult. Mentioned here are only a few to give you an additional sense of the wide impact toxicity has on elder services. They are the Information and Assistance (I & A) and Ombudsman programs under the AAA, plus the Hospice program.

Information and Assistance

I & A phone counselors receive a wide variety of requests pertaining to multiple problems from diverse callers. Toxic agers are among those callers. Nevertheless, most I & A counselors become skilled in maintaining their patience and sensitivity to toxic agers. For example, one veteran advisor commented,

> Toxic behavior is a cry for help, although they'd [the toxics] never admit it. It's just that their anger and resentment have built up for so many years, they need someone to listen to them. True, they do take up a great deal of our time as they call repeatedly, but we listen as much as we can, and tell them to get active and get out of themselves even though they probably shun our advice.

Toxic agers are generally very resourceful in using every means at their disposal to quell the anxiety within and to feel noticed. When they run out of face-to-face contacts, they will resort to phone services. They are desperate, lonely people.

Ombudsman Service

Also under AAA, ombudsworkers manage cases that involve older adults in institutional settings. Their goal is primarily to empower residents under the Patient Rights Act and to follow up on complaints. They are the patient's advocates, mediating numerous problems and issues that range from health care to fiduciary and legal issues, family intervention, and providing adequate facilities. Much of their work concerns putting out fires. They do not have the staff or the training to give in-depth, long-term social service.

Like other service providers, ombudsworkers face multiple issues, both mental and physical, toxicity not excluded. The following will illustrate how toxic agers can have an impact on service providers and interfere with attempted care. One worker called it "a job for getting flack."

> Another ombudsworker (I'll call her S) stated that she had had at least 40 or 50 toxics in her caseload over a 10-year period and that 30% to 40% of those appeared to be deserted by their families. As the daughter of a toxic father she could understand how the adult child of a toxic parent might feel. To illustrate, she spoke of one daughter who faithfully called her father and paid all his skilled care bills but was unable to handle a personal visit.

Still, looking back, S conceded that it took her several years before she could work through her own experience with her toxic father and be able to "detach" professionally. She exclaimed, "Until I learned how, I would either burn-out or become a bureaucratic basketcase. Toxics can literally kill us, if we let them." Now S uses her personal experience and knowledge to create workable tools for coping (see Part IV).

S did remember one case, however, about 5 or 6 years before, in which she had no solution. The Medi-cal patient was a female "Southern Belle," married five times, with no relatives except a nephew and his wife. Claiming that the nephew's wife stole her property, the patient (I'll call her Belle) caused all attention to be focused on possible fiduciary abuse. It was some time later before the staff discovered that Belle hated any woman who had a "man." It was a 20-year vendetta. Meanwhile, the unbearable situation caused the nephew and his wife to move to another state without giving anyone their address or telephone number. "It was as if they dropped off the earth," said S. Even moving Belle to a small, all-female board and care home did not work because Belle was then all over the young man who came in to help.

Hospice

In this case, the hospice MSW was assigned to a 75-year-old male who had been an operating engineer building the Alaska pipeline. Although declared legally blind, he had been living alone in a small, filthy trailer that had not been cleaned, including removing the trash, in 16 years. The patient spent his days smoking, listening to the radio, and distressing everyone. According to a neighbor the client had been argumentative, suspicious, and difficult for many years. His physical diagnosis was congenital heart failure. He could get some relief by being on oxygen, which he continued to use while he smoked. He refused assistance with bathing and denied having any family. He trusted no one and did not believe the hospice worker when she said she wanted to help him maintain his independence and thus needed some information on his finances. He replied, "It's none of your business."

The patient did share that when he was a young boy his father had left the family "high and dry" and that later, when the patient's mother was sick, he stayed and cared for her after the other siblings left. Apparently, the patient never had a sense of anyone caring for him, acting oblivious, as he aged, to his desperate surroundings. There had been a marriage, but it was shrugged off, dismissing all women. Finally, a sister was located who said the patient owed her some money and that she was the custodian of his bank account.

Death came soon to the patient, seemingly anxious to be released from life. Left behind, however, was a hospice social worker (one who knows how to be professionally detached) distressed over the condition in which she found her patient. Was it the patient's toxicity that shut him off from help? Probably. We don't know. We do know, however, that it had an impact on a seasoned social worker.

Multiple Issues—Differential Diagnoses

Clear differentiation between toxicity and other diagnoses may be difficult at times, especially if a history is not obtained, because surface symptoms will sometimes appear to be similar. In the following cases there are either dual or multiple diagnoses. Recommended practice is to treat the presenting problem first. Recognition and consideration of the impact of toxicity on the treatment, however, is imperative. If ignored, toxicity will definitely obstruct treatment.

Alcoholism

In sharing experiences with alcoholic agers, it was obvious to several caseworkers that toxicity and alcoholism were meshed. As one worker commented, neither toxics or alcoholics

> can live within the family, can be placed in adult day care, or keep homemakers. Both refuse services until they are desperate. Then if they do accept help, they only become argumentative, complain excessively, and are nonappreciative.

Both toxics and alcoholics can also be smooth con artists. Manipulation is a mainstay. It serves them well in hiding the way they treat their children from the service provider. Their sweet talk is sometimes hard to resist. One caseworker explained that when she was forced to close a case after there was nothing else she could do for the client because all resources had been exhausted, the alcoholic simply found another sympathetic ear and the case was reopened. This continued, on and off, every 3 to 6 months until the agency ran out of susceptible workers, an example of the Big "R" Rescuer game pattern referred to earlier.

Multiple Medical Diagnoses

Described here is the case of an 80-year-old mother and her daughter. Mother has multiple diagnoses of mild to moderate vascular dementia, diabetes, hypertension, osteoporosis, and depression. Daughter has been in a support group for 6 months, monopolizing the group's discussion with problems with her mother and the underlying issue that she was molested by her mother as a child. It appears that both mother and daughter are toxic, with the daughter also becoming the client.

The only other source of support for the mother was a financial contribution from the ex-spouse, who was estranged from both mother and daughter. The mother did have two brothers, but they were both alcoholic and no help. The mother insisted she was not an alcoholic, which soon became suspect when some of the memory test results came back normal.

Mother was referred for partial hospitalization because she was not taking her medications (often found on the floor), dressed inappropriately, was found naked outside, and, when shopping, would walk out of the store, leaving the grocery basket half filled. Her toxicity usually erupted in power struggles with the daughter when the mother continuously refused all treatment, including a conservatorship. Utterly frustrated, the daughter was finally hospitalized for an attempted suicide.

It took months of continuous work on the mother–daughter relationship before the LCSW involved could help the daughter bring her mother in for lengthy assessment tests and treatment and work out some joint strategies for helping them both learn how to function together, despite the mother's perseverance in a domineering control role. Initially, the daughter was afraid to even phone the mother about her appointments because the mother's anger and resistance to treatment were always vented on the daughter.

When the worker intervened, typically simple therapeutic procedures evolved into challenging and taxing sources of frustration. One technique employed by the social worker, just to get the mother to come in to the office, was to let the mother think she had seduced and charmed the worker into thinking there was nothing wrong with the mother. This was accomplished by endless listening and praising, plus acceptance of the mother's home-grown tomatoes at each visit. In time, however, these attempts to reach the mother became excessively time-consuming, putting an additional strain on the social worker while the mother's pervasive, manipulative noncompliance tactics continued.

At the end of our interview, the LCSW wearily said, "This case has taken an inordinate amount of time and resources. I'm feeling overwhelmed and drained," feelings aggravated by the mother's multiple calls each day and the lengthy voice-mail messages left at night. Even in the parking lot, the worker could not avoid the daughter. She would park her car next to the LCSW's car in order to catch the worker and "talk." The layers of problems made the therapy and medical treatment unnecessarily difficult.

Working with two advanced toxics can be unbearable if one cares too much. "How much time can one give to one case?" sighed the social worker.

Mental Health Disorders and Toxicity

Two geropsychiatric cases will be discussed here: one hospitalized and one who refused hospitalization for 7 years.

The initial case was an 89-year-old toxic female diagnosed with a major depressive disorder. After the pain from her degenerative arthritis and bone disease was relieved, the patient's negative energy was fully released. She focused on criticizing and belittling other patients and refused to follow any goal-directed treatment. In a resentful tone, the daughter of the toxic ager lamented, "She's always been that way."

According to the MSW on the case, the hospital "had lots of toxics," and the patient immediately found other "crankies" she could get along with. It seemed that they delighted in engaging each other in putting everyone else down.

Initially, remembering some of her experiences with her own toxic mother helped the MSW with the case, but being new to the job, she tried hard to impress her boss and get both his approval and that of the client. Consequently, she found herself depressed, anxious, and feeling incompetent when the toxic patient did not respond. For awhile she thought something was wrong with her, until she recalled her studies on countertransference. It was a difficult lesson for the social worker. Eventually, her patient did begin to respond. She became more open and directable, allowing others to begin to support her rather than chasing away any intended help.

In the second case, a 68-year-old (undiagnosed at the time) bipolar manic-depressive, toxic female resided in a residential facility in a large urban county. Physically healthy and attractive, she walked 4 to 5 miles daily and consistently refused any thought of psychiatric assessment.

The client reached the attention of ombudsman services because she incessantly complained about every residential facility she was in. Treatment was always inadequate, her clothes were either ruined or stolen, the staff was uncaring, the doctors did not take care of her properly, and it was all Howard Hughes' fault. He started it by ruining every relationship she ever had.

At first the ombudsworker, who started out as a part-time volunteer and had been on the job for only 2 years, was convinced she could help this woman. For 5 years the worker tried. There was little improvement. The client was moved from one facility to another. Nothing changed. Discontent and criticism of residents and services was a consistent pattern. Finally, after placing the client in the last facility available in the county, the worker called mental health, only to be told there was nothing they could do to help. By now the client's complaints had extended to calling 911, 15 times a day and writing the district attorney to inform him that nothing was being done to help her.

Finally, in total frustration one day, the ombudsworker told the client, "There's nothing else I can do for you. You have to help yourself" and walked out. She immediately called a coworker to take over and left the case.

Within a few weeks, however, the client called back, begging the original worker to continue to work with her. This time the client was willing to listen and agreed, after 7 years, that she needed help. She was later admitted to a geropsychiatric unit and diagnosed, another example of how the insecurity and fears of losing control can effectively block a toxic's care and treatment and torment a service worker.

Toxic Spouse and Brain Impairment (Alzheimer's Disease)

An especially difficult situation, this case was assigned to an MFCC consultant and specialist in family support care. Involved were an elderly brain-impaired wife (the presenting client), a toxic male spouse (the caregiver), and a supporting daughter (an only child).

The family toxicity showed up when the trauma of the wife's Alzheimer's disease set in. Denying her loss of memory, she exhibited paranoid behavior. Whenever she could not find something, which was often, she accused others of stealing it. Fearful and confused, her anxieties were exacerbated by her spouse's verbal and emotional daily abuse. Consequently, outsiders were reluctant to enter the home to help.

Although not brought to the attention of social services, the spouse had a long pattern of toxicity. Typical of many elderly toxics, it did not become an external, or public, problem until the wife's illness disrupted his long-standing patterns. With the advancement of her condition, the husband's fear of loss of control was intensified. Not trusting anyone, he refused to cooperate with the MFCC. His expectations were unreasonable. He was demanding and domineering, and because of his perfectionist orders and standards, no one could please him. Although the counselor finally got the husband to agree to hire professional respite help, 3 days was the maximum a helper would last. He either fired the caregiver or they would leave, unable to take his constant harassment and criticism.

The spouse also refused to allow his wife to go to adult day care, saying "Oh, she's fine at home." Like all toxics, he was good at playing the martyr role, that is, until the care got to be too much and his tolerance ebbed. That was when he would phone his daughter and demand that she drop everything and come over immediately to take over. This included many calls at 4 A.M., after he had been up all night with his wife and could not get any sleep. The daughter would dutifully respond, only to be put down and criticized after she arrived. She could never do anything right. At one time the father was so upset with his daughter that he forbade her to see her mother for 6 months, a display of the inner, conflicting turmoil toxics experience.

Over time, the drain on the daughter became visible. She had numerous chronic medical problems and lost her job when her father's demands caused her to take too much time off from work. This led to a loss of income and eventual eviction from her apartment because she could not pay the rent. Depressed and on the verge of a nervous breakdown, she felt her life was a shambles.

Although deeply concerned about the outcome of this case, the MFCC had to admit she was relieved when she learned the family had moved away. She still thinks of them, and I suspect shudders at her own sense of helplessness. She was not used to that kind of outcome, yet with the husband refusing any help, there was nothing else she could do. The family's toxicity and dynamics were too enmeshed. Any attempted group work or traditional therapeutic approach proved futile. Still, the situation was not serious enough to be taken over by APS. It all seemed so hopeless.

Caregiver Support Services

In the early stages of toxicity, most agers do not involve the services of a professional caregiver. Help is sought only when the toxic symptoms are compounded by physical or emotional degeneration, medical needs, or dementia. Problems can arise quickly for caregivers, however, if they are not trained to know what to expect from toxicity and how to handle it. Because the role of the caregiver is constant, consuming, and demanding, it is difficult to sustain permanent help if the caregiver can never do anything right. As one daughter exclaimed,

> Mother has gone through six caregivers in 2 months. She always finds something wrong, then fires them on the spot. She doesn't even tell me what she's done. I find out the next time I go to visit. I'm at my wit's end. I don't know where to turn.

It is especially important for home health aides and other caregivers to receive training not only in what to expect and how to deal with and understand the toxic patient, but also in how to protect themselves from the toxic's demeaning attacks, blaming, and game playing.

Daughters who begrudgingly take on the caregiver role out of desperation, guilt, and duty especially need training or they will invariably become co-Victims. Unless the daughter shifts her perception of the role, she is vulnerable. As a caregiver, she is now on the receiving end of a daily barrage of negative energy and behavior. She bears the brunt of constant manipulations, projections, displaced aggressions, and other defense mechanisms and psychological games, as well as being overly susceptible to the unconscious seduction of the toxic hooks. The phrase, it is safe to attack family, truly applies here. There is no letup until possibly the latter stages of dementia when the internal emotional torture of the toxic begins to dissipate.

As with Alzheimer's disease, toxicity is an ultimate stressor and will break any untrained caregivers, especially if they are themselves needy helpers, or *Rescuers* (see Karpman's Triangle in chapter 10).

Strong words? Yes, but hopefully they will jar us into looking honestly at a painful reality. Toxicity can destroy the spirit unless caregivers, professionals, and families recognize that it is a masked cry for help and calls for "tough" love.

Pitfalls in Caregiving

Trouble occurs when professional caregivers have a felt need to "make the patient happy." New caregivers particularly delude themselves if they believe they have this kind of power. Trying to "make" anyone happy, especially a toxic, is masochistic. Likewise, giving advice or taking on the role of a parent only leads to bad feelings and endless frustrations that invariably evolve into anger, guilt, and distance. The relationship then disintegrates, and both the caregiver and the receiver become Victims.

If the decision to become a professional caregiver is made with the full knowledge of what to expect and how to deal with it, caregiving can be very meaningful work. Nonattachment while maintaining a caring mode is a critical balance. When achieved, there is no clinging to false hope or anticipation of gratification for services rendered. It is realistic attending and professional.

Residential Care

According to one experienced social worker employed in a facility with 85 residents, most residents have some form of dementia. Many are also toxic. An example of a situation that frequently has an impact on the staff was related. It occurs when husbands who have been caring for their toxic wives die. The children (if father has not protected them from their mother's toxicity and dementia) know their mother cannot be left alone. Consequently, immediately after the funeral the children move mother into a residential facility and then leave, often permanently.

Meanwhile, the staff is left to deal with mother who, by this time, is confused, fearful, and crying out, "Where's my husband?" The caregivers try to reassure the mother, calm her anxiety, and explain what is happening, but the combination of toxicity and dementia dissipates all effort. Little helps. Furthermore, the staff does not have time to listen to the mother's endless whining or deal with her attention-seeking clinging. They are forced to focus primarily on looking out for her safety and her medical or physical needs.

By this time, the other residents have also experienced the mother's toxic behavior. They refuse to associate with her or sit at her table. To defend herself, she outwardly proclaims, "I don't care. I like being by myself. That's their problem." Then the paranoia sets in. In one case, the mother accused everyone of stealing her lower dentures. She now has the attention she needs, but she's still alone.

Retirement Communities

Despite their active and happy-looking appearances, large retirement communities also have toxic agers—many if you talk to the social workers. Two examples are offered to depict how toxic agers can have an impact on the professionals, especially if they are children of toxic agers.

> This situation centers around a long-term, independent living, self-sufficient toxic resident in her early 80's. It was recounted to me by a social worker consultant, trainer, and group facilitator with years of experience in the gerontology field.
>
> It seems that the toxic woman involved (I'll call her B) was at one time president of the senior council of this particular retirement community. The council's task was to oversee and coordinate the activities, rules, and other matters dealing with the members. Although B was no longer an officer of the council, she still considered herself head of the organization and behaved as if she was totally in charge. Often she would walk into the director's office and demand

an immediate response. An issue was made about anything that was not the way B wanted it.

B constantly told people off; had no regard for others' feelings; blatantly insulted, attacked, and criticized; and then vehemently objected to any feedback about her own behavior. In the council meetings B would disagree with the decisions, loudly interrupt others' comments, push her opinions, and literally disrupt every session. Other members complained incessantly about B but never to her face. They just gave her a wide berth.

In desperation, the new president of the council finally contacted the social worker (I'll call her Z) for help. Z learned what she could about the group and its dynamics, then attended their next meeting. Making her presence known, Z watched the proceedings with care. Suddenly things got out of hand. B was yelling at the president who, red in the face, was now yelling back. As it escalated, others joined in. For the first time in her professional life, Z felt she had lost control. She put her arms up across the door and shouted, "No one is leaving this room until this is settled." The scene was tense. Z said she did what she could, then walked out.

Following that episode, if Z encountered B, B would turn her back and "huff off." She refused to talk to Z. Instead, B spread untruthful rumors and stories that would have damaged Z's professional reputation if believed. Attempts to confront B only made the situation worse.

Not used to this degree of toxicity, nor her own loss of control, Z was disturbed. It had never occurred to her that as the daughter of a toxic she was particularly vulnerable to the toxin and thus susceptible to countertransference. Because she was unaware of what was happening at the time, Z instantly hooked into B's behavior. Any nonattached professionalism dissolved. Instead, Z perceived B as having no redeeming qualities or realness, of employing cunning ways to be ingratiating, and of being the "greatest bitch she had ever met."

Here is a situation in which the toxic ager B becomes (symbolically) Z's own toxic mother, causing Z's hurt inner child to unconsciously employ its own projection identification defense mechanism onto B in an attempt by Z to ease and avoid dealing with her own emotional pain.

It was years later that Z shifted her perception of the incident and could see the situation and the toxic older woman differently. The shift did not come easily. It followed many months of intensive personal work and training in Byron Katie's exercises and teachings known as "The Work," a process described in chapter 13. The Work awakened Z to her own toxicity and helped undo her negative internal beliefs through perceptual shifts and an unconditional self-nourishing love that started the healing process.

A sign of Z's transformation was revealed when she finished her story to me and said quietly, "Today, I see B differently. She is the saddest person I've ever met."

Another experienced LCSW at a large retirement community proclaimed, with instant irritation in her voice during my initial call for an appointment, that there were "too many toxics" at this community and that working with their defective character disorders was "unrewarding, draining, and frustrating; and if not careful, could lead to a hardened, displaced bitterness." Then, just as suddenly, there was dead silence. After a pause, and in a much softer voice, she said. "I'm so burned out right now, let's get together when I get back from my vacation."

Listening to herself and recognizing her own exhaustion and overextended schedule, which included no time for self-nourishment, was a smart professional response. Hearing the defeatism and anger in her voice, I readily agreed to the delay. We met 3 weeks later.

It was some time into the interview before I learned that the social worker (whom I'll call M) had a toxic mother and a toxic grandmother. The impact was telling and definitely influenced M's going into the gerontology field.

Growing up, M had watched the effect her grandmother's toxicity had had on M's mother. It seemed to be the catalyst that compelled M to teach as many caregivers and adult children as she could about how to prevent this type of behavior from having an impact on them. Focusing on the parent-child relationship, how to cope, and how to understand the dynamics of the interaction, M's professional load expanded to conducting classes for intern caregivers and facilitating group work for children of toxic older adults. Her goal was to become an independent consultant and conduct workshops specializing in toxic agers and family relationships.

M went on to relate one example of the kind of thing she watches her mother experience over and over when dealing with her mother, M's toxic grandmother.

M describes her grandmother, at age 95, as cute and with only a mild impairment considering her age. In describing her mother, M sees her as emotionally overinvolved and abused as she tries, futilely, to please the grandmother. The daily pattern consists of M's mother calling the grandmother to offer to do or get something for her.

In a recent situation, the grandmother asked M's mother to pick up some ibuprofen, when it was convenient, for her arthritis. Fine, no problem. No problem, that is, until M's mother walked in with the pills and grandmother threw an immediate tantrum, belittling and criticizing M's mother for not using the 50-cent coupon that was in the newspaper that morning. Having no awareness of the coupon, there being no earlier mention of its existence, plus receiving no thank you or any gesture of appreciation, the outburst leaves M's mother feeling inept and discounted—again.

This type of interaction is repeated routinely between the two women, vividly demonstrating the toxic loop cycle and some of the unconscious transactions that I call co-Victim games. Some of these games are "Look What I'm Doing For You," "I'm Only Trying to Help", "Gotcha," and "Poor Me" (see chapter 10).

Assessment. Does M's never-ending exposure to toxic behavior affect her? Unquestionably. Interestingly, M responded to her mother's toxicity the same way I did to my own mother's toxic behavior. The impact on both of us was so wrenching that it led to a professional determination to help others avoid the same kind of pain. To do this we searched for information. We sought ways to learn more about toxic behavior, to understand its dynamics and what caused it, and to see if it could be prevented and treated. For M, working with a combination of toxicity and mental illness was like "having a client from hell." She needed answers and had already done considerable research to attain them.

M's specialization is centered on the relationships between older parents and their adult children, as evidenced by her recommendation of Secunda's book, *When You and Your Mother Can't Be Friends* (1990). M's emphasis includes a focus on maladaptive behavior, marginal coping of older adults, the differences between what M calls "the great Depression and immigrant mentalities," and the subsequent conflict therein between mothers in those eras and the baby boomers who are working and have different values and expectations. According to M, unable to fulfill the perceived care expectations of their mother's generation and being raised in feminist thought that implies you can "do it all," care-concerned daughters are torn between guilt over what they believe they should be doing to help and what is realistic. Trying to do it all is certain burnout, something M understands only too well.

The Depth of Toxicity Impact

As portrayed, adult children who are vulnerable to toxicity in a parent are deeply affected, despite professional status and knowledge. Transgenerational passage is common to those susceptible, regardless of training. Perhaps this can be best illustrated by sharing my own experience and awakening to the toxicity long denied within me.

The first time I became aware of my own toxic trappings was the countertransference experience mentioned earlier in this book during my initial research interviews with toxic agers in 1989. The second time was after the editors' review of the first draft of this book early in 1997. The review reflected an overall tone of anger throughout the manuscript, a disowned, unacknowledged anger that accounted for a sizable loss of objectivity and, subsequently, a total rewrite of this book.

I was aware that toxicity often exposed itself when least expected and usually without conscious awareness. Learning, however, that I was not as healed (or recovered) as I thought I was was a jolt to my perceived sense of self. This revelation, although difficult to accept at first, was another opportunity for growth for which I am now deeply grateful. The anger in me—my own toxicity—was so deep, so buried, so hidden, so repressed that just acknowledging it was not enough. Besides, I thought I had worked it through. Now I know my toxicity is part of me and will continue to involuntarily erupt in a multitude of unexpected ways until I can free the unconscious fears and shadows with unconditional self-love.

With emotional understanding, I can now truthfully say I know the anger that unconsciously drives most toxics, an anger—and the fear underneath it—that can be disallowed throughout a lifetime. It is often terrifying and begs for healing. It takes time. For us aged toxics, even recovering ones, surveillance will be ever constant.

Summary

This chapter describes and assesses the impact toxicity has on professionals and service providers in the gerontology field. Because toxic old and old-old agers are found in all aspects of the field, professionals from a wide spectrum of services were interviewed. The general feedback is that up to now, professionals were basically left to their own resources in devising ways to cope with, and manage, emotionally abused and abusive elders.

In facing reality, many examples are presented from a variety of areas and types of problems confronting these professionals, how they are personally affected, and their subsequent inability to give the kinds of services they desire in order to meet the needs of their toxic clients.

To make the examples of toxic cases, and their impact, easier to access, they are organized into categories and subgroupings: new caseworkers, senior centers, public services, private practice, special services, multiple issues and diagnoses, residential care, and retirement communities.

Represented are services contracted through AAAs, such as Ombudsman, Home Health Services, and I & A, plus those offered by the Public Guardian Office, Hospice, and APS, as well as those addressing multiple issues related to toxicity and alcoholism, differential medical diagnoses, and mental health disorders.

Also included are special cases that depict the impact of toxicity on professionals who are also children of toxic agers and the sense of helplessness counselors can feel when faced with a toxic caregiver spouse, his wife with Alzheimer's disease, and a daughter who is unable to please either.

I hope these examples will help you, the service provider, have a greater understanding of the impact of toxicity on professionals in the field of aging.

Chapter 6

Potential Co-Victims?

You may be wondering why there is a chapter on co-Victims and others on whom the toxic ager has an impact. It is simple. Co-Victims and significant others are the key to treating toxicity. True, it is possible for professionals to instigate some temporary behavior change, but with toxics it is only a momentary cover so they can continue to get what they want. It does not help them face their deep fears, anger, and shadow parts of themselves.

Care providers and significant others, such as spouses and adult children, can make a difference by changing the way they respond to toxic elders. If the family system and dynamics are disturbed, the agers will be forced to do something different just to feel safe. It is one way to break through their defense barriers and induce a need for change. If the breakthrough does occur, healing can begin from within, but only if the toxic ager makes a conscious choice to change. External single efforts by the family or caregiver will only give the abuser's ego another opportunity to maneuver into a new control-cover and prolong, enhance, or perfect a new psychological game.

Because care providers are critical to the instigation of the toxic's healing process, it is important for significant others to be included in the treatment, either as advisors or co-clients. Some of the cases from the last chapter exemplify the fruitlessness of working strictly with the toxic ager as the sole client. Understanding the impact toxicity has on those closest to the client, and how his or her responses and perceptions need to be shifted in order to alter the system dynamics, is consequential. In addition, the *degree* of game interplay involved needs to be assessed in order to focus adult children workshops and training sessions appropriately. Because it takes at least two to play these psychological games, teaching significant others how to stop their involvement in the toxic loop is probably the best approach with toxic agers and will be discussed in depth in the section on TA in chapter 10.

How Does Co-Victimization Happen?

In the definition of toxicity in chapter 1, I stated that toxicity was a character maladaptation that produces a negative energy of Victim consciousness. To clarify this further, this negative energy is contagious for anyone who may be susceptible, including professionals. This means they unconsciously allow themselves to be pulled into the toxic games and become potential co-Victims.

Although the negative energy can be felt just by walking into a room, co-Victimization does not occur unless there is a mutual, albeit unconscious, willingness to play the toxic game. If an unaware player is *hooked*, the game can replay interminably, without the coplayer consciously knowing what is happening. Without awareness, professional position, power, or traditional training are useless. Adult daughters, themselves vulnerable to the passing on of toxicity, are the most susceptible.

Distinguishing Between Difficult and Toxic Clients

Before you can teach others about toxicity, you will need to clarify for yourself the difference between difficult and toxic clients. Practice discernment before you label them. Like toxics, difficult clients are also frustrating and taxing, but if your interaction does not involve a negative feeling that totally drains your energy, it may not be toxicity. A toxic game transaction leaves a penetrating, bad feeling that is unmistakably felt and is a clue to be noticed. This distinction is critical. Just because an ager cannot get along with others, is stubborn and refuses to listen, habitually does things that push your buttons, or is simply irritating or different does not necessarily mean that he or she is toxic. Difficult does not translate into co-Victim. Toxicity does.

Also noticeable is the difference in the degree to which people respond, or hook into toxic behavior. Out of 20 professionals, there may be only 1 or 2 that succumb to the toxic game. Out of a family of four children, however, at least one may become a full-blown co-Victim. Reasons for this behavior vary as much as the variations in individuals. I know of no study that empirically documents the cause. In my own work, however, I have observed that personality type seems to be a factor. Individuals who compulsively need to please and be needed, but disregard their own needs, and are excessively helpful but guilt prone, appear to be the most vulnerable to the co-Victim syndrome (see the Enneagram in chapter 8).

Clues to Watch for

When individuals do fall into the co-Victim trap (professionally called countertransference) they will sense everything from a vague, inexpressible negative feeling and energy drain to the following explicit symptoms:

- Emotional exhaustion
- Guilt and frustration
- Resentment or anger
- Depression
- Overimmersion in the other's problems
- A sense of being cheated out of a nourishing, normal relationship
- Futility in trying to please
- Never being able to do anything right
- Excessive dutifulness or obligation

- A feeling of being "stuck" and helpless
- Sadness or despair
- A feeling of being victimized

Why the Focus on Co-Victims?

When working with toxic clients, traditional counseling or psychotherapy is counterproductive. It is not business as usual. The toxic's resistance and noncompliance will block most of your efforts. Find the co-Victim. There always is one; it takes two to play the toxic game. He or she may be the key to any kind of progress with the toxic if you are able to perceive and work with him or her as a coclient.

When the co-Victim client is willing, teach him or her the coping and change strategies described in chapter 12. Set up support groups. Let the members hear and learn from each other. Spend the time. In the long run you will have affected multiple families, broken the generational cycle, and helped a toxic ager.

How Does Toxicity in Agers Impact Others?

The others referred to here include staff and professors at a college institution, adult children, spouses, friends and neighbors, and grandchildren who have also experienced the impact of toxic agers.

Impact on a College

Usually only a small percentage of 70- to 85-year-olds are found in a formal educational setting, and even fewer of these are toxic. If a toxic ager has no friends and no family, however, a community college can easily become his or her life. Yet, as desperately as they need the school, toxic agers will continue to practice their uncanny ability to push people's buttons with almost every contact.

From personal experience as a college counselor working with reentry and older students, I spent many hours one year doing damage control with admission officers, deans, department chairs, teachers, and clerks having to deal with just one toxic ager (I'll call her T). T's scowls and her loud, harsh, piercing voice, which accompanied countless unreasonable demands for immediate service, were common. These demands were not only annoying, disruptive, and time-consuming, they also interfered with services to other students.

In time, the irritations become so stressful to those on the receiving end of the toxicity that they threatened to file formal complaints with the Dean of Students. They wanted T disciplined or, even better, expelled. Rarely, however, was any direct effort made. How could one justify the expulsion of a 76-year-old? And on what grounds? Besides, as was typical of most people dealing with toxic agers, no one seemed willing to confront T personally.

Finally, the limit was reached in one department in which T kept repeating classes. Unable to tolerate her disruptions, her inability to handle the content of the classes, and wanting to avoid her anticipated complaints to the Board of Trustees, extensive maneuvers were initiated by the department chair to get T to drop out. Program designs, grading systems, the number of times a student could repeat a class, and the use of part-time teachers were all revised just to get T out of the department and prevent others like her from enrolling. It took considerable effort, many meetings, and more than a year of hassling bureaucratic systems, until it was finally accomplished.

It seemed unrealistic to believe a little old lady could so intimidate everyone she touched, but it worked and had for years. It was rare to find any professor or staff member able to confront T directly. Even grades by a part-time teacher, fearing her complaints, were inflated, prompting the part-timer's dismissal when it was discovered.

Resolution. In follow-up interviews with the chair of the besieged department (I'll call her C), who had instigated and maneuvered the changes to manage students like T, it was obvious that C was deeply distressed. The troubles had spilled over into C's home life, and there were many hours of cathartic listening by her spouse. It was not until I learned that C's mother was also toxic that I understood some of the dynamics of C's misery. Although an exemplary professional in her field, C had never faced, or been able to cope with, her own mother's toxicity. T's presence had brought it all back. T became C's mother, and once again C's unresolved early pain and anguish were unconsciously experienced and projected onto T. She became a co-Victim.

It wasn't long before T moved on to another department, her third. Fortunately, this time it was discovered that T had a natural gift for the requirements of that department. She could excel and was accepted. The professor had been previously briefed on the situation; understood and agreed to take on the challenge; solicited the other students' help; and gave T special attention, encouragement, and support. (The other department chair had tried to do so but had been rejected by T.) In time, T's class disruptions, outbursts, and inappropriate questions and comments diminished.

Only one minor change in the classroom procedures was made. Students were required to make regular critiques of other students' work. Therefore, a policy was established that before the students could give critical feedback, they had to say what they liked about another student's project. Apparently, T's critiques were just too harsh, pointed, and sharp, one of her skills. It was affecting the other students and undermining their sense of ability and self-worth. The structured format helped shift the perception and demoralizing projections.

T was fortunate. The school became the place where appropriate social skills could be taught (when she was willing to accept them) without focusing directly on her and triggering her fears and defenses. Is this the role of a college, however? If naive and unaware of the fallout of toxicity, how can it avoid becoming a co-Victim? Is the disruption of the system worth the time and effort and the taxpayer's money?

Impact on Adult Children As Care Providers

Adult children are the ones most likely to be affected by toxic agers. Their newly acquired position of care provider forces them into frequent contact with elderly parents, regardless of the nature of their previous relationship, often after many years of living apart with separate lives. Children are taught to "love, honor, and obey" their parents, despite the circumstances. Negative feelings toward them are repressed, and any association with toxicity is hidden. You just don't discuss it.

Usually, it is one adult daughter who becomes the care provider of a toxic parent and the child most affected. She is also the one who becomes the co-Victim. She is either left with the responsibility or feels so duty bound by her values and personal feelings of "oughtness," that she assumes the role. The impact on her can be devastating.

From personal counseling, workshops, and support-group feedback, I learned that the effect of toxicity not only leads to depression and resentment, but that most of the involved daughters of toxic agers are in psychotherapy. My concern was heightened while listening to five of them talk. One daughter admitted, rather hesitatingly, that she had contemplated suicide. Immediately, three of the four others present said they had also considered suicide. I realized then that the impact of toxicity was even more serious than I thought and needed to be brought to professional and public attention.

To aid in bringing the seriousness of toxicity to light, I have included the following comments from the adult children's feedback and personal interviews regarding their toxic parents.

She's so controlling!

She's probably getting worse as the family is never honest with her. We just reinforce her reality.

I feel sad (and guilty) that I do not love her.

After 34 years, I realized how destructive my relationship with my mother was. I guess I'm a slow learner, but it took that long to understand that there was *no way* I could make her happy or please her!

My relationship with my father seemed so cold and distant. Only once do I ever remember his putting his arm around me. Why didn't he ever tell me he cared?

I'm constantly amazed. She used to be exceptionally kind to others. Always volunteering with some charitable organization. No one would believe how she is at home.

I feel so burdened. She is so ungrateful! I try so hard. Nothing I ever do is right.

She's so blind to what she's doing to others.

It really woke me up when my college-student daughter said she wouldn't come home for Christmas if Nanna was there.

The whole family has tried to confront her. It is not worth the effort. It just made her more impossible, more hysterical, more enraged. We've learned the best thing to do is just get away, if possible, and avoid the outburst.

Sometimes I'm so full of anger.

Adult Children As Caregivers

Attention also needs to be given to the single adult child left with the daily parental support. Other adult children, neighbors, and acquaintances can walk away. Professionals and caregivers can leave after a set time or limited hours, but the adult child who takes on the full 24-hour responsibility and perceives that she or he *has* to always "be there" for that parent, including the endless, around the clock phone calls, is bound. Day and night, weekday or weekend, the demands and disruptions continue. Torn between family responsibilities and his or her mother, there is no personal life left.

This type of mother–child interlock is a common reality. Many daughters and sons are already hooked into the Rescue game (see chapter 10) and codependency. There are personal and psychological reasons for this, but few explicit and certain answers.

Even if we understand the causes, it does not alleviate the penetrating emotion felt by the involved adult child, an emotion she or he may not even be able to identify. Inside is a vague angst that, if examined, is called fear. It is a deep feeling that especially announces itself in a daughter's frequently heard, bitterly expressed, words:

> "I never want to be like my mother!"

The telltale words of a daughter of a toxic mother.

Unless we have experienced the situation, we cannot fully understand the depth of anger and fear in those words. We cannot feel it or comprehend the accompanying bondage. The involved adult children of toxics, in order to heal themselves, must awaken to the reality of their predicament. They must acknowledge the truth. Avoidance only buries the anxiety until it festers. Whether they like it or not, they *are* like their parents.

Fear of toxicity is real. Studies of abused children have taught us that abuse seeds abuse. The victim eventually becomes the perpetrator. In this way, toxicity is unwittingly passed on through the generations, stopped only if the destructive pattern is interrupted.

Compulsive and thoughtless remarks that unconsciously spew out of our mouths at our own children make stopping the pattern without help doubtful. With a haunting feeling, we notice that these are the very words we vowed we would never use on our own children. We are not even aware of what we do until we look back, analyze the situation, and recognize the displaced aggression defense mechanism. As a parent we may have momentarily protected our own ego illusions and maintained our self-esteem, but to vulnerable children, the damage is done. Yes, the old saying is true, "We hurt the very ones we love the most!"

Aware toxics regret this type of compulsive behavior but are seldom able to stop it, or prevent its eruption, without constant effort. Negative habits become so ingrained that repressed feelings break out into endless, unconscious overreactions to even small, insignificant, daily incidents. Family members become the scapegoats, the "safe" outlets. Children on the receiving end of toxic behaviors, such as irritability, perfectionism, blaming, and constant complaining, are its negative legacy. Professionals can be the intervening force to break the cycle (see Part IV).

Impact on Spouses

I suspect that the major difference between the way spouses and children survive the toxicity of an aging member of the family is the manner in which they distance themselves from the perpetrator. Until adult children are forced into the caregiver role, physical distance is effective for the children. It is usually not an option for a spouse.

Spouses must deal with the toxicity on a daily basis and often over a long period of time. Most of them experiment until they find coping techniques that will work. Unfortunately, too many spouses of the older generation prematurely conclude that their only option is simply to learn to "live with it." This decision is made because the thought of divorce, getting the other to change, or coercing him or her into therapy is inconceivable. Feelings and "dirty linen" are not to be aired in public.

Also, the toxic behavior may have crept up so slowly over the years that the spouses are not cognizant of what they are dealing with and often unable to identify the destructive patterns. They simply adapt to the behavior or have learned through sad experience that any attempts to modify it are futile. Instead, we often see passivity and repression of feelings, a withdrawal defense.

Older male spouses often find it difficult to even discuss, or admit, a toxic situation. It is easier to block out the behavior, ignore it, or avoid it. As one husband professed, "I've learned the hard way. That's the only way to get along with her." For him blocking it out may have worked, but such a relationship essentially evolves into a strained habit.

Avoidance Examples

Such strained habits were evident during the latter half of my own parents' 53-year marriage. Seven years my mother's senior, my father retired and died while she was still working. For years I watched him progressively withdraw as her toxicity worsened. Daily job separation made it possible for them to endure each other. Healthy confrontation was inconceivable. They could not face a relationship that had become toxic for them both.

I doubt if my mother ever realized why my father pulled away into his own world. When he buried himself in his newspaper, magazines, books, yard and carpentry work, a loud TV, and excessive sleeping on the couch to avoid her constant complaining, whining, and fault finding, his behavior was only annoying to her. To him, however, it was a way to slow down the outbursts, and it did, but the negative vibrations never lessened.

The depth of toxic entanglement in spousal relationships usually depends on the value system of both partners, their particular propensity for toxic game playing, the duration and extent of the toxicity, and the process used to contain the dysfunctional behavior and response patterns, especially before retirement. After retirement, the constant, daily contact forces attention to the toxicity. Some families can deal with it; most cannot. Usually the persons involved have no concept of what is going on, what is wrong, or what to do.

> In another long-term marriage, the toxic was a 73-year-old, lifelong alcoholic female. Boundaries were blurred between her toxicity and her alcoholism. Because she was also physically impaired and could not go up and down stairs, the husband fixed a room for her on the first floor with her own TV and other comforts. He then had his own room and TV on the second floor, where he spent as much time as possible to get away from her whining and moaning.
>
> When the social worker visited, the wife complained bitterly that her husband totally ignored her and would not come when she called.
>
> On the surface, this could have been perceived as a case of elder abuse and neglect if the social worker had not questioned further and learned that the wife was referring to one incident that occurred at 3:30 A.M. The husband had simply not heard his wife.

In dealing with toxic cases, it is important for you, as a professional, not to jump to conclusions or make assumptions but to listen carefully and ask comprehensive questions that will lead to accurate assessments. Complex issues do not have simple solutions. Plus, be constantly watchful. With toxics, there is usually a co-Victim.

Impact After Retirement

Several female spouses in long-term marriages with toxic agers were interviewed. The women proclaimed that their husbands were good providers and had had many virtues in the early years of their marriage—before retirement. Their toxicity and need for control was tolerable earlier because it had been constructively redirected through jobs that required them to be in positions of power. These men often worked long hours, as well as being occupied with activities outside the home, such as community boards and commissions, or became absorbed with their children's activities. They directed plays, taught Sunday School, supervised camping trips, or coached youth sports.

When the children grew up and the community and work-related activities ceased, and there were no plans for the psychological aspects of retirement, there was nothing left to reinforce the false self-image and need to control to which these men clung so desperately. Worst of all, they had few friends and no support system. To them, being vulnerable, a requirement of love and friendship, was not allowed.

> Another example of toxicity after retirement was the husband who had been an exceptionally skilled bridge player. One evening while playing bridge, he realized he could no longer remember *all* the plays of the game. Despite the fact that even with some memory loss he was still better than most of the other players, it was not good enough for his self-imposed perfectionist standards. Because he could not control the situation and others would see his weakness, he could not bear the shame. He was too inflexible to change or adapt and could not express his feelings or ask for what he needed, so he simply quit playing, hibernated, and wallowed in his own self-pity.

> In another example, a counselor in the gerontology field emotionally severed the marital relationship with her toxic husband in order to survive and maintain her own mental health. In her late 60's, she built a segregated life for herself through her work, community involvement, volunteerism, and friends. To an outsider, things looked normal because the couple continued to live in the same house. In actuality, however, they had separate rooms, separate identities, and lived separate lives. It was a long-term marriage retained only for economic necessity.

These are additional examples of the creative resources on which individuals closely associated with toxicity can draw if they refuse to become co-Victims. There are coping skills and practices you can encourage as you work with co-Victims.

Husband Cover-Up

Male spouses affected by a toxic elderly wife sometimes use a cover-up tactic with children who live out of town and visit infrequently.

Whether consciously or unconsciously, the father intends to protect his adult children from their toxic mother. By intervening, making excuses, or taking the blame for difficult situations, he controls the interactions. "He'd be the brunt," as one daughter-in-law put it.

Because of their father's interference, the adult children seldom have any idea of the daily frustrations and energy drain experienced by their father. Many older men do not want to bother their children with their problems. "We can take care of ourselves," they boast proudly, wanting to be strong and not show their feelings. Consequently, the adult children hear only, "Everything is just fine. Don't worry about us." Dad gets away with his cover-up. Inevitably, however, perhaps on his deathbed, the final words would come: "Mother is not the easiest to live with. Just be patient with her. Take care of her."

The subsequent shock is not easy for the children, and it falls to the professional to ease the crisis and teach the adult children, especially the care provider, how to cope.

Impact on Friends and Neighbors

According to the circumstances and type of relationship, the impact of toxic agers on friends and neighbors varied. The irritations and "put-up-withs" ranged from small daily incidences to time-consuming efforts to help, especially if the toxic ager was female, in poor health, and lived alone. Most friends and some neighbors were willing to help as much as possible, at first, until they were "used up." Many, however, soon become frustrated and exhausted and ended up either shunning the toxic elder, doing as little as possible, or even calling the police if things got desperate.

One exception was found. In this situation the toxic involved had been a next-door neighbor for 20 years, even baby-sat the children. When her husband died and she was left alone, the toxicity became visibly evident. The neighbors, responsible, caring people who remembered how she used to be, just accepted the situation as part of life. Initially, they took turns fulfilling the frequent demands of their toxic neighbor so that no one in the family had to carry the load. Despite the best of intentions, however, the teenage son seemed to be left with a major share of the work. This was attributed to his skill in not only being able to humor his toxic neighbor, but also not "hooking in" to her games, manipulations, and demands. He became the neighborhood stabilizer when others had "had it."

Impact on Grandchildren

Because toxicity is usually passed down through the generations, grandchildren can be uncommonly perceptive in assisting potential co-Victim Moms to "wake up" to their own toxicity. Helpful feedback is quick if Mom simply asks, "Please, will you be willing to make a contract with me to let me know whenever I act or sound like Grandma? I promise to listen and not lash back at you if you specifically alert me to what I'm doing that may be toxic."

Called a Contract in TA, this is a strategy that not only helps Mom as the care provider but also educates both her and the grandchild about toxic behavior patterns, explicit honest communication, and how to cope and avoid being "hooked" in to the toxic games and becoming a co-Victim. It is also another teaching tool (see chapter 10).

Grandchildren Feedback

The grandchildren of toxic agers interviewed ranged in age from 17 to 39, with an average age of 26. Responses varied from those whose relationship with their toxic grandparent was nonexistent to those who simply ignored their presence, those who acted polite and "shined them on" (tried to please), and those whose tears flowed heavily when they talked of a once-loved grandparent. Many were still working through their grief over the loss of an idol, friend, and model.

All the grandchildren interviewed seemed eager to talk, as if to say, "At last there is someone who will listen and maybe even understand what I've been going through!"

As the interviews progressed, it became apparent that although the stories varied in particulars regarding the way each person handled his or her situation, there was a common thread. The disruptive, repellent behavior of a toxic grandparent was pushing the grandchildren away from a relationship that had often been cherished when they were young. Back then, grandma gave them attention. She was somebody, in their childlike minds, that they could look up to. As time went on, however, it became obvious to them that many of the family problems that had been occurring were caused by grandma's toxicity. The grandchildren could feel their parents' pain and empathize with their agony. They had begun to understand, and even recognize, some of the same symptoms in their care provider mothers.

As they matured, most of the grandchildren managed their feelings and thoughts by maintaining some distance between themselves and their toxic grandparent, interacting as little as possible, even when grandma lived close by. Phone calls were sparse and dreaded. Only 2 of the 17 grandchildren interviewed stated they felt they had learned to cope with the situation and didn't "let Grandma get to them." Nevertheless, the pattern was consistent. Visits became fewer and fewer, occurring only when forced by parents.

To give a personal sense of the impact of toxicity on this third generation, some of their thoughts and feelings were compiled from their responses to interview questions.

1. When did you first realize that your grandparent was toxic?

   According to one grandson, "She was always controlling, argumentative, and self-centered. My concerns intensified when I got my own children."

   "Just the past couple of years. Now it's getting out of hand. She's negative most of the time. I didn't sense it before. I'm not sure if it's because she's getting older, or if it's because I can see it now."

2. How does your grandparent's toxicity affect you emotionally?

   "I won't let it. I usually get her involved in something or change the subject. I won't let her drag me down."

   With tears rolling down her face, this granddaughter described being hurt and upset. Feelings of anger also arose when she explained how her grandmother had refused to see her 7-month-old great-granddaughter, even though the baby was named after her. She exclaimed,

"I can't understand it. I was the closest, and until I was 12, my grandmother took me in on weekends so I could get away from my father. We were *very* close. We even shared secrets. I could tell her all my problems, and now she won't even talk to me. I really want to be part of her life. I want to be liked by her."

"I felt irritated with both my grandmother and mother. For awhile it was tough as I took over and was in the middle, but now I'm pregnant, and I can't handle it anymore. Besides I have to think of my own family."

"I'm really tense and apprehensive, guess you might say drained and angry. Every time I talk to her, I'm afraid I'll say something wrong."

"It has contributed to my low self-esteem. I'm also bothered as I see how it has affected my mother."

3. Describe the behavior that you consider toxic in your grandparent.

"The negative attitude, the mopey withdrawal, the bitterness, the belligerence, the depression, the lack of tact. For example, her pronouncement that now that she is old she has the right to 'tell it like it is,' regardless of who it hurts."

"She's constantly blaming others and will never admit to anyone that she is wrong."

"She's always complaining and criticizing. You can't do anything right, plus, she never forgives you. Then she wants you to be constantly in her life, yet in the same breath she's pushing you away."

"She's so rigid. Everything has to be her way. You've got to go by the rules, *her* rules. And if there's a disagreement, she's not interested in working things out."

"She's constantly badgering us. She confuses love with gifts and favors and then expects twice as much in return. If you don't do something for her, you don't love her. If she doesn't get what she wants, she goes screaming to other members of the family and starts pitting us against each other—just creating trouble until she gets what she wants. And she usually does."

"She always wants attention and gets upset if she doesn't get it. She even uses illness to prevent others from leaving her. Or, she complains about all the work she has to do, then refuses to accept any help. Also, she'll pick fights with her husband, with my Dad, or anyone that's not neutral. You can't have an opinion in her house unless it's her opinion."

"She teaches you to lie in order to avoid an argument or an outburst."

4. Describe your greatest fear regarding this situation with your grandparent.

"That she will hurt someone that loves her" (said with tears in his eyes, making it clear it was not himself he was concerned about).

"Losing Grandma before she and I can patch up what we've lost."

"That I'm going to blow up and scream at her, and she'll have a heart attack, and I'll be to blame."

"I fear there will be more damage to my mother. She's already overstressed, and then she overreacts."

5. Do you perceive your grandparent as aging normally?

"I don't know. I don't know what it means to age normally."

"No, because my other grandmother is not like this. She's mellow and accepts life. And my friend's grandmother is sure different."

The depth of perception of these grandchildren is clear. They can be a vital support in changing the family dynamics, interaction system, and toxic games.

Is Toxicity Progressive?

All the grandchildren interviewed said they felt their toxic grand-parent's behavior had gotten progressively worse with age. They also admitted that it was possibly more noticeable because they themselves had become more aware. Several said it was more apparent after the death of their grandparent's spouse, job loss, stroke, breast cancer, or some other traumatic event.

Can Toxicity Be Prevented?

When asked if they ever confronted their grandparent about his or her behavior, most of the grandchildren visibly shuddered. Faces filled with fear, followed by an "are you crazy?" look. Yes, there were times they would yell and lash back when grandmother was out of control, but confront her assertively? With love and understanding as the focus? "You got to be kidding?" What an absurd idea!

For some grandchildren, the idea of rationally confronting their grandparent was never an option. A few had considered it, but it just wasn't something you did. Besides, there was no point. It was sheer futility to confront their feelings or behavior. The repercussions would be too great. Besides, their grandparent would deny everything anyway and then blame someone else for all the problems. They knew the pattern. It was simply best to avoid any kind of conflict at all costs, and avoid is what these grandchildren did, whenever given the choice.

What Happens to Toxic Agers in Public?

Most of the grandchildren interviewed expressed amazement at the difference in how their grandparent responded to others in public, especially with strangers, clergy, and some social workers. In public (unless the degree of toxicity was well advanced or severe) their grandparent would turn on the charm, the manners, the consideration, and the highly honed manipulative skills. Out-siders rarely believed the truth about them. Without visible toxic behavior why should anyone believe the family? In defense, silence became the practice. Truth was rarely expressed. Like most dysfunctional families, the syndrome became hidden and remained hidden until the toxic behavior affected others and could no longer be buried or ignored. By then, however, it was often too late for intervention.

Is Toxic Behavior Justified?

Most of the grandchildren felt that toxic behavior was not justified. To them, no excuse and no explanation could justify the way their mother or father was treated by their toxic grandparent. One grandchild did feel sorry for her toxic grandmother but admitted that the pity she felt did not make for a good relationship. Other grandchildren were disgusted with the "Poor Me" pity games displayed and the habits that only further separated everyone involved.

Summary

Why write a chapter on co-Victims? This chapter is important because toxicity creates Victims. It is almost as if they coexist. Therefore, it is crucial for professionals in the field of gerontology not only to plan on working with the co-Victim, but also to see him or her as a co-client, and as an asset in helping the aged client. It takes at least two to play the toxic game (see chapter 10); therefore, if the co-Victim changes or stops playing, the interactive system changes and the game stops. The toxic ager, in turn, is forced to respond differently in order to maintain his or her psychic equilibrium. Understanding the co-Victims, and to what extent toxicity has an impact on them, is fundamental in working out a plan of action.

Also examined in this chapter are a number of questions. How does co-Victimization happen? How do people allow themselves to be pulled into toxic games, especially the professional who may be the child of a toxic parent? Can we discern the difference between the difficult client and the toxic client? What kind of clues do we look for? If the co-Victim's consciousness is raised, so that he or she can be taught to stop the toxic game, will that end the toxicity at least in the aspect of passing it on to the next generation?

Then there is the question of why different responses to toxic agers either deter or encourage the behavior. Examples of case situations are given pertaining to college personnel; adult children and their role as caregiver; spouses and their avoidance habits and other coping tactics, the impact after retirement, and husband cover-up; friends and neighbors; and the grandchildren and their perceptions and feedback regarding questions such as the following: Is toxicity progressive? Can it be prevented? What happens to toxic behavior in public? Is toxic behavior ever justified?

I hope the preceding information will help you devise your own support team for working with toxic agers and avoid becoming co-Victims.

Part III

What Causes Toxicity?

It is the theory that decides what we can observe.

—Albert Einstein

Chapter 7

Can Theoretical Research Explain Toxicity?

Toxicity in aging is not new. What is new is the name "toxic," its association with the aged, and our concern about identifying the cause or causes of toxicity.

In any search for answers, particularly regarding a specific behavior, the same questions invariably arise. Is it nature or nurture, or both? Is it genetics, the environment, or a combination of these?

These questions form the basis for the organization of Part III of this book. Gerontological research, and my own studies and theories, will be addressed in this chapter. Subsequent chapters will include other literature review arranged in the following categories:

1. Personality: focus on inborn typology
   Is Nature the cause?
2. Environment: significant other influence
   Is Nurture the cause?
3. Script Maintenance: keeping it all going
   Is it Nature and Nurture?

Approaches: Two different types of research are used to distinguish some statistical indicators of toxic behavior and the abstract postulations of theories and concepts.

1. An empirical study of data obtained to differentiate successful agers from the unsuccessful (toxic) agers.
2. A literature review of gerontological, social, and psychological theories and models that could show links to the cause or causes of toxicity.

Empirical Indicators of Toxicity

In my original research (Davenport, 1991), a comparison study was made among 44 randomly selected, matched subjects age 64 to 86, questioning why some older adults aged successfully and others were unsuccessful (now referred to as toxic).

It was discovered that although the unsuccessful toxic agers had less money, inferior housing, inadequate education, perceived (not actual) poorer health, and more religious ritualism as compared with the successful agers, the data were statistically not significant.

In contrast, data found to be significant at the 0.01 level revealed that the unsuccessful toxic agers had

- Defective coping skills
- Inadequate interpersonal relationships
- Few to no intimate friendships
- Deficient support systems
- Little outside involvement
- Minimal resourcefulness
- Insufficient physical exercise
- Negligent eating and health habits
- Self-orientation to the past
- More confinement (few drove cars)
- Lived alone longer
- Self-centered tendencies

- Refused to acknowledge their fears
- More dependence on outsiders
- Dwell on negative events

Although helpful in identifying behavior, these data appear to be indicators, or symptoms, rather than means to clarify any specific cause, or causes, of toxicity.

Therefore, we might assume that these symptoms are only the effects of toxicity, not the causes. But what do the symptoms tell us? Many of them are present in each of us to some degree. Why do they get worse in only some agers? How do they affect the aging process? Why do some older adults age so differently, even though their life situations and personal circumstances are similar? Is toxicity one of the reasons people differ in their aging process (Davenport, 1991)?

I soon discovered that I was not alone in asking these questions. In studying the literature, I found that the developmental psychologist, teacher, psychoanalyst, and author Erik Erikson and his wife Joan (while in their 80's) had been asking the same questions. In the book *Vital Involvement in Old Age* (1986, p. 55), written with Helen Kivnick, they wrote,

> How is it that one individual may seem able to *integrate* [emphasis added] painful conditions of old age into a new form of psychosocial strength, while another may respond to similar conditions in a fashion that seems to inhibit effective integration and healthy, ongoing development?

Davenport Theories and Hypothesis

It is hoped a review of the literature will uncover clues to plausible causes of toxicity, and that the theories and models examined will provide a framework for exploring and building new responses and workable interventions. But first, I want to propose my own hypothesis and theories that are pervasive throughout this text.

First, it is my theory that most of us are caught in a world produced by our own perceptions, a world governed by our own thought processes—those learned, selective, unstable, and often inaccurate interpretations of internal and external input. We see and hear only what conforms to our wishes and self-distortions. It is a world that reflects our internal belief system, not the facts. It is a mirror of ourselves, a *perceived reality* that is only an illusion, not truth. In addition, it is our choice.

This concept of choice is pervasive throughout *A Course in Miracles* (1975). According to its premise, we choose our own state of mind, how we want to live, and where we want to feel safe. Our mind reflects the fearful nature of our own self-image and the prison we have made to contain it.

These prisons become our lifestyle, our way of being, determined by how we interpret our emotional and mental states, values, previous experiences, ego needs, expectations, childhood conditioning, and relationships. They are the consequences of how we organize our internal and external signals. They bring into being the defense mechanism we call projection, a tactic whereby we attribute to others and the environment what we admire or despise in ourselves. It is a subconscious, habitual pattern that accomplishes well its ego-protecting purpose but is destructive to open, honest relationships (Davenport, 1991).

Projections can be positive or negative, self-deceptive or factual, painful or joyful. They become the basis for judgments, decisions, actions, and a false worldview that only exists in the minds of the perpetrators. A life pattern is formed, with the projectors unaware, and not responsible, for what they have made.

Analogy

For instance, if individuals perceive the world as morally bad and full of hatred, pain, and attack—and the self as the helpless victim—they are fooled into believing that this perception is the truth. With it as their reality, they can justify their frustration, negativity, anger, paranoia, and fear, but uneasiness still remains.

The ego, fearing its own vulnerability and need to control, entices its victims with quick defense solutions that not only ease the momentary pain but also protect the ego's own existence while it deceptively returns a feeling of personal power to the victims. Unaware of what is happening, this illusion of power gives the victims a renewed sense of control and safety, and, once again, they fall into the ego's trap. Habitual response patterns are formed and played out continuously. Troublesome as it may appear, this is the world Victims make and cling to, the world and pattern of toxic agers.

Scenario

To illustrate the preceding, let us imagine toxic agers who, imprisoned by their ego, perceive themselves as losing control and their sense of security. Fear sets in. They are terrified. They are getting old, losing their personal power as well as self-identity. No one comprehends their inner desperation. Even they do not understand the disquieting feelings they are experiencing. Where do they turn? They turn to the past and the ego, futilely hanging on to old, now-dysfunctional, childhood coping skills and the ego's relentless defenses.

Unaware that they are also grieving over their perceived losses, these toxic agers get stuck in bitterness and anger. They see themselves as victims. In fear, they unconsciously lash out, projecting onto others (usually their family) the very things they despise and fear in themselves. Feeling bad, guilt is now added and projected back onto the family. Eventually, a cyclic habit and a toxic worldview of distorted illusions, twisted perceptions, defenses, and control mechanisms are set in place. The toxic loop becomes more and more rigid.

Based on these assumptions and theory, the following hypothesis was developed:

Individuals consciously or unconsciously *construct* [emphasis added] their own reality and lifestyle in response to how they perceive, interpret, identify with, give meaning to, and define internal and external environmental signals. (Davenport, 1991, p. 6)

Gerontology Theories

Of the many gerontological theories, I have focused on the Continuity Theory and the work of Robert Atchley on Discontinuity as most pertinent to toxicity.

Continuity Theory

Long considered one of the most inclusive theories of gerontology, Continuity Theory has been discussed and debated by gerontologists since the 1960s. Some claimed it to be the most promising theory in aging (Covey, 1981; Dreyer, 1985) because it was in the framework of the life-span perspective and a component of Activity Theory. Successful aging, under Continuity Theory, was considered the continued development of an adaptive process for balancing our life course and roles in accord with our own preferential pattern and personality style as it fit accustomed, and socially structured, restrictive role expectations.

Gerontologist Robert Atchley (1972) probably described it best:

> Continuity theory holds that in the process of becoming an adult, the individual develops habits, commitments, preferences, and a host of other dispositions that become a part of his personality. As the individual grows older, he or she is predisposed toward maintaining continuity in his or her habits, associations, preferences, and so on. (p. 36)

Undoubtedly it is this continuity of lifestyle that James Birren, gerontologist, editor, and professor, referred to when speaking at a conference on *"Aging and Wholeness in Later Years"* (1987). Birren said that "stability was one of the two features that emerged from the many studies on adult personality, and lends itself to the interpretation that in general we become more like ourselves with advancing age" (Birren, 1987, p. 31).

If we define personality as the predictable way we perceive ourselves, others, and life events—and our response patterns coincide with that perception—it follows that a stable continuity would emerge (Reedy, 1983). Likewise, it would seem that if this perception is warped and reflects a dysfunctional lifestyle pattern, a similar dysfunctional pattern would also emerge (Reichard, Livson, & Peterson, 1968).

It was Atchley, however, who brought the negative side of continuity (the nonnormative and dysfunctional, although predictable, aging response patterns) to the attention of the gerontology community when he first identified it (1989).

Discontinuity Theory

In labeling his new theory "Discontinuity," Atchley proclaimed that there were some agers who were unable to employ strategies they had used in the past, that these strategies were no longer effective in helping the agers cope or adapt to the changes of normal aging, or that the agers never had effective coping skills to begin with. Discontinuity and stress occurred when their perceived internal and remembered identity was in conflict with the perceived external structure of their new roles, activities, relationships, and environment. Pathology would then occur, and normal development was impeded.

Atchley further stated,

> The standards used to assess continuity reside in the personal constructs used by the individual to organize his or her perceptions. People construe the world around them by means of a personal repertory of concepts and it is this personal repertory, which may include social constructions of reality, that guides decision making and evaluation. These personal constructs are organized, often nonconsciously, into a theory of how the present is linked with both the past and the anticipated future. (1989, p. 185)

Note the similarity of Atchley's thinking to psychocybernetics (see chapter 10) and the basic hypothesis of this book: Individuals consciously or unconsciously construct their reality according to internal and external perceptions of environmental signals.

Thus it stands to reason that an aging toxic person who persists in clinging to outdated, internal perceptual constructs because he or she is unable to adapt, accept, or cope with the natural changes of aging will not attain the desired stability expressed by Birren (1987). Disorganization, discontinuity, and distress follow. There is a "tilt" in the automatic response system. Subjectively remembered, internal images, those interior pictures that once gave a sense of self, security, and ego protection, are in conflict with the toxic's external reality. This is not the self the toxic perceives himself or herself to be. Unless the internal and external constructs and images can be reconciled, integrated, and healed, dysfunction continues and normal development is blocked. Defenses only intensify. This is *not* successful aging.

Atchley did not call agers in discontinuity "toxic," but it appears he was referring to the same phenomenon.

Once again we see attention paid to the power of perception relative to the way individuals order or disorder their own reality and life structure. When things are not consistent, when they are out of balance and past response patterns no longer work, disorder is the feedback, inner disturbances are the experience.

Invariably, the questions rise again.

1. How do we cope with these forces?
2. Can the conflicting inner pictures, constructs, and perceptions be changed?
3. What coping skills can be introduced to replace the excessive use of old defense mechanisms and bring back continuity?

Summary

Part III of this book concentrates on the search for the causes of toxicity in aging. This chapter examines research literature, theories, and data; identifies exploratory questions; and outlines the organizational structure of the other three chapters to follow the major issue of whether the cause is nature or nurture, or both, and how the toxicity is maintained.

The search for answers is divided into two approaches: (1) an empirical study of toxicity indicators and (2) a literature review of pertinent social, gerontological, and psychological theories.

Empirical data revealed a significant contrast between the unsuccessful toxic agers and the successful agers in the study. Although the data indicated only behavioral symptoms, it can provide some directional clues for further research regarding possible causes of toxicity in agers.

In addition to examining the concepts that form the working hypothesis for this book, a review of the gerontological theories of Continuity and Discontinuity were also considered. Atchley's Theory of Discontinuity is especially pertinent because it professes a nonnormative, dysfunctional, negative side of a predictable aging response pattern.

Chapter 8

Is Nature the Cause of Toxicity?

Is it possible we are born with a tendency to be toxic?

Typology theorists would say yes we are born with innate personality tendencies, traits, and preferences that are a key to human behavior. Good or bad, they are dictated by our own special genetic codes.

Life-span developmentalists, on the other hand, would argue that it is the environment that shapes and forms the personality and subsequent behavior. Others, such as myself, believe that personality is a combination of nature and nurture, that selective, response choices of environmental stimuli and perception can build on, or suppress, nature's inherent givens.

In this chapter personality-type theories will be examined as possible genetic factors in the causation of toxicity.

Personality Definitions

To facilitate a common frame of reference when speaking of personality, the following definitions are presented. Most professionals would probably agree that personality is a set of predictable response patterns, character traits, and qualities that when presented to others socially define that individual. Typologists would probably add that it is the set of inherent preferences and tendencies that uniquely shape the way individuals perceive and interact with their environment.

These perceptions can also evolve into a false self, an ego illusion that is manifested in a predictable set of response patterns and character traits whose interactions are formed by internal self-perceptions of early experiences, expectations, motivations, values, and self-image. These response patterns can then be detected by the way they are projected onto others, a self-mirroring.

For example, if the self-perception (as with toxics) is contaminated and built on misinterpretations, negative messages, and low self-image and esteem, toxic individuals can easily become fixated at a low level of development and project these self-hate perceptions and distrust onto others. If that happens, successful aging is doubtful. Instead, the deceptive image, or false self, becomes another critical ingredient in the shaping of a complex toxicity syndrome and an unhealthy personality type.

Personality Theories

Although the literature abounds with personality theories, there are four that I want to emphasize. Two studies were developed by gerontological life span researchers, one through an ancient oral tradition called the Enneagram and the last based on Jung's personality type theory.

Gerontological Theories

Study One

As far back as the 1960s, some gerontologists considered personality type to be one of the keys to successful aging and a variable in how people respond to life, whether they respond with satisfaction or dissatisfaction. In 1967, researchers such as Reichard, Livson, and Peterson identified five personality types based on a study of 87 men, ages 55 to 84 years (Turner & Helms, 1979). From the most ideally adjusted to the least adjusted they labeled these types as (1) mature (constructive), (2) rocking-chair (dependent), (3) armored (defensive), (4) angry (hostile, blaming others), and (5) self-haters (self blaming or depressed).

The first three types were considered to be well-adjusted. They behaved and interrelated in accord with their perception and acceptance of themselves in their earlier lives. The last two were easily frustrated and characteristically depressed, developing a predictable lifestyle commensurate with their self-perceptions, again strengthening the basic hypothesis of this text.

Study Two

A year later, Neugarten, Havighurst, and Tobin (1968) reported a similar classification based on their 6-year Kansas City study of several hundred elders age 50 to 80. Four personality types emerged. They are:

1. *Integrated.* Well-functioning, flexible, acceptance of "impulse life," over which they maintain comfortable control, open to stimuli, and demonstrate high life satisfaction.
2. *Armored-Defended.* Achievement-oriented, ambitious, striving personalities who positively use their defenses to maintain their need to control impulse life and thus attain functional life satisfaction.
3. *Passive-Dependent.* Exhibit a continued lifestyle of dependency and nonassertiveness with lower levels of satisfaction.
4. *Unintegrated.* Low both in activity and life satisfaction, labeled the *disorganized*, persons whose thought processes show deterioration, have no control over emotions, and are psychologically defective, although maintaining themselves in the community.

With the results of these early studies, patterns of aging appear to be consistent with early behavior unless there is an intervention to create change. Values and characteristics become more salient as individuals choose how they are going to interact with their environment, with most toxic agers falling into the last category.

The Enneagram

Probably the most applicable personality typology system available to help individuals understand toxicity and its possible causes is the Enneagram. Pronounced "any-a-gram," it is an ancient trans- personal system for understanding human nature. Based on East- ern wisdom and using a nine-pointed diagram, the system divides humanity into nine core personality types. These are connected by maplike lines that form a directional path for healing. Since the Enneagram was introduced to the United States in the early 1970s, it has evolved into a Western psychosocial-spiritual system for self-development, business applications, and journey into wholeness. The breaking of its oral tradition in the mid-1980s brought an explosion of books—more than 50 between 1990 and 1995 alone—distributed worldwide. So we ask, can the Enneagram answer the basic question of aware toxic agers: "Why do I do the things that I do . . . the things that I would not do?" As an energy system, can the Enneagram explain what drives toxics?

Because of the Enneagram's subtlety, complexity, and sophisti- cation, it is best approached at three levels.

- *Social Level:* to accept, understand, and respect differences in self and others and their impact on interpersonal relationships.
- *Psychological Level:* to acknowledge and release compulsive dysfunctional behavior, ego-fixations, negative defenses, and self-deceptive illusions in order to enhance self-development, embrace the shadow*, become vulnerable, and be open to transformation and wholeness.
- *Spiritual Level:* a *spiritual awakening* whereby ego control is transcended, where true essence, the higher Self, and the healing power of Divine love and grace are found.

Resources

Given the multiplicity of the Enneagram, only a broad overview can be presented. For the history and a more thorough understanding, review the authors named in this chapter. Key also are G. I. Gurdjieff, Oscar Ichazo, and Claudio Naranjo, who were instrumental in introducing the Enneagram to the United States.

For beginning students I recommend Baron and Wagele, *The Enneagram Made Easy* (1994) and *Are You My Type, Am I Yours?* (1995). For the more advanced student there are *Personality Types: Using the Enneagram for Self-discovery* by Riso and Hudson (1996) and the audiotape by Palmer (1995). For the therapist, *Transformation Through Insight: Enneatypes in Life, Literature and Clinical Practice* (Naranjo, 1997), describes Naranjo's character-oriented and ego-style conscious therapy called "Enneatype-conscious gestalt."

The Essence of the Enneagram

A few of the early teachers and authors of the Westernized perception of the Enneagram are quoted here to offer a sense of its potential in understanding why the constructs of this personality typology system relate to toxicity.

For Helen Palmer (1995), in the Introduction to her audiotape series, the Enneagram is based on centuries of mystical traditions and esoteric practices of ways to

> shift the negative pole of the personality to its opposite tendency . . . to discover the motivation within yourself that is the *passion* [emphasis added] or negative tendency, and through psychological insight and understanding, or the spiritual methodology of meditation, to interrupt the automatic habit of the passion so it doesn't express itself and cause damage to others in the environment.

To Hurley and Dobson (1993), the Enneagram's purpose is

> about unity within oneself and among human beings. It's about healing the hidden pain of life. It teaches how to release the power and creative energy to follow one's destiny, and through it to discover what gives life. The Enneagram is about soul making. (p. 17)

Therefore, it can teach how to prevent and intervene in the making of a toxic and his or her co-Victim.

Richard Rohr proclaims in his book *Enneagram II: Advancing Spiritual Discernment* (1995, pp. ix, x) that the Enneagram "is a powerful spiritual tool . . . a conversion tool for the transformation of consciousness. There is no way through it without the experience of abandonment to grace. . . . It is primarily food for the soul."

For Rohr, Ephesians 4:22–23 says it even better:

> You must give up your old way of life, you must put aside your old self which gets corrupted by following illusory desire. Your mind must be renewed by a spiritual revolution. (*Jerusalem Bible*)

What Is the Enneagram?

Diagrammatically, the Enneagram is a geometric symbol consisting of a nine-pointed star and specific connecting lines, all enclosed in a circle (Figure 8.1). Each point on the star represents

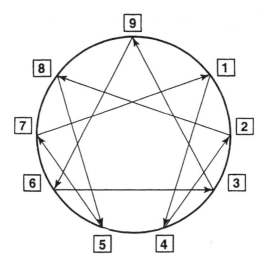

FIGURE 8.1   The Enneagram symbol.

one personality type. The term "Enneagram" comes from a combination of two Greek words: "enneas" meaning nine and "grammos" meaning a measuring unit or point (Brady, 1994; Hurley & Dobson, 1991).

Structurally, each Enneagram point has an assigned number that represents different energies and patterns of self-deceit, ego-fixations, illusions, avoidances, fears, passions, and virtues. Each of us carries a part of all nine Enneagram-type energies within us, but one of the types is an innate preference and the controlling dominant force from which we design a life blueprint pattern, or *life script* as TA would call it. Within each point is a wounded spot, or place of opportunity, from which we learn to develop and balance our strengths and gifts, unless we distort them beyond the balance and they become "have to" compulsive behavior. Without the attention of self-observation, these unexplained compulsions can slide down the connecting lines into unhealthy, toxic behavior.

The arrows in the Enneagram diagram represent the particular paths and directions to travel when things are going well, or when there is a time of distress. As such, the arrows are a guide to a state of psychological health, thus becoming an added tool for prevention and early intervention work with potential toxics. The numbers on each side of the core type number are called Wings and also influence the manifestation of each type (Beesing, Nogosek, & O'Leary, 1984; Keyes, 1990; Palmer, 1988; Riordan, 1975; Riso, 1990, 1996).

The Enneagram's Significance to Toxicity

Formed in a symbolic circle of life, the distinction of the Enneagram's innate personality identification is that each particular core type position is based on motivation and perception, not behavior, and therefore might indicate the causes of negative behavior. Movement around the circle into unified wholeness is the goal.

Because each Enneagram type responds differently to distress and trauma, familiarity with the personality system helps professionals differentiate which approach is the most effective for each type. For instance, type One perfectionist toxics, especially older ones, fear loss of control and will criticize, find fault, and attack until they have a sense of control, feel safe, and things are again "right" according to their perception. Distinctions among each core type can help professionals understand and work with the varied core differences and toxic responses.

Why Is the Enneagram Considered a Powerful Tool?

The power of the Enneagram comes in its ability to

1. jolt the self-deceptions and ego illusions;
2. provide a map for individuals to travel on a journey of discovery as to who they are;
3. transcend traditional psychological models and address and integrate the social, psychological, and spiritual components of wholeness and emotional health;
4. particularize the path for each personality type's healing and personal growth;
5. aid in the identification of the level of unhealthy or healthy development or energy;
6. help in the understanding of "why" we do what we do, consciously or unconsciously;
7. understand the annoyances of symptomatic behavior;
8. encourage the embrace of the shadow in order to heal and break dysfunctional habits and fears;
9. lead to a true essence and inner peace, if one is willing, and able, to make the journey; and
10. show us how to find love, the missing ingredient in the lives of toxics.

Early Enneagram Premises

George Ivanovitch Gurdjieff was the first to use the Enneagram in Europe in the late 1920s. According to Gurdjieff (Tart, 1983, 1986), the basic concept of the Enneagram states that human beings are asleep and locked into a system that fosters illusions of self-deceit, especially as it pertains to the concept of who they are. Because the points of the Enneagram are interconnected and oriented to movement, individuals can uncover more about themselves by looking at the direction in which they choose to move within the system, a choice that can be helpful or hurtful, positive or negative. If the choice is positive, individuals become balanced and move toward wholeness and integration. If the choice is negative, as with toxics, they simply fall deeper and deeper into their toxicity and pathological layers until they are caught in the endless feedback cycle as described by *cybernetics* (see chapter 10).

Enneagram Personality Types Most Susceptible to Toxicity

During my interviews with toxic agers, I noticed that two Enneagram personality types seemed to show up with more regularity than did the other types. Their predominance left me uneasy. They were the two patterns and Enneagram numbers with which I was the most familiar—my own. The first was my core type, known as Type One (the Perfectionist). The second was Type Two (the Helper) and my preferred Wing. At first I was shaken. Some of my deep suspicions regarding toxicity in my own family were being confirmed. Professional curiosity was stimulated and a deeper, more persistent search for possible causes of toxicity ensued.

As a daughter of a toxic ager, and having been raised in a toxic environment, I had already started to face some of the natural fears of being or becoming a toxic ager myself. Undoubtedly, this contributed to my immersion in this work. Knowing this, however, did not ease the uncomfortable feelings that now penetrated my very being. I knew how long I had already worked on my own, unhealthy toxic tendencies. I also knew why they were so difficult to change. Although I despised the behaviors, they were mine, and I had to "own" them, not get rid of them.

It has taken years of determined effort just to reach the point of acknowledgment. The unwelcome response patterns I created are deeply rooted in my sense of identity, attention, and security. They are a way to structure time that becomes a lifestyle, but, worst of all, they are governed by my unconscious, my defense mechanisms, and my ego. They have become, to my chagrin, an *addiction*.

Enneagram Type One. Some of the major issues, struggles, and imbalances of the Enneagram type One—the toxic-prone perfectionists—are incessant judgmentalism; repressed anger at inequities, injustices, and imperfections in the world; unreasonably high standards; and the compulsive driver inside that says they *have to* make things right, but right according to *their* perceptions and standards. Add to that another type that is the most prone to be the co-Victim in the toxic game, my Enneagram Wing Two (the Helper), and we see an intense person carrying the weight of the world.

It was my preferred Two Helper Wing that trapped me initially when my mother became my responsibility as a declining old person. That unhealthy Two part of me constantly fell into the entanglement game of "Look What I'm Doing For You," "Poor Me," and "I'm Only Trying to Help." It was my Two passion of pride that compelled me to help, to the neglect of my own needs. At the time, however, typical of all Unhealthy Helpers, I did not know what my needs were, nor was I aware that I probably avoided them in order to be a martyr. It was always "yes" to the other person, unbearable guilt if I wasn't helping someone in need, or the endless failed attempts for 34 years to please my toxic mother and try to *make* her happy.

Not surprisingly, society praises both the Helper and the Perfectionist for their efforts, never realizing the cost to the individuals. Perfectionists are achievers and self-starters. They work hard, are reliable, maintain morality and integrity, and always seem to be cleaning up or straightening out others' messes. They are good people but, like all examples of Enneagram points, they have a dark side. Few outsiders know that underneath the One's smile is a resentment, an anger, that is avoided and feared (good girls and boys do not show their anger). This avoidance leads to excessive scorn for emotional weakness and control of themselves, their environment, and everything in it, just to feel safe.

When distorted and out of balance, the One's gift of goodness tends to be moralistic and rigid, leading to toxicity. Unhealthy Ones vociferously let others know if something isn't "right" according to their unyielding, unrealistic standards. This includes fussing and complaining about everything from a crooked picture on the wall to an unethical advertisement, a flaw in a sentence, someone not following through on what they said they would do, or something the toxic thinks somebody else should be doing but is not. It is constant. In a toxic One the words are out before he or she is even cognizant of what was said.

Trouble arises when toxic-prone people age and the rules change. Now it is time to release their controls, adapt, be flexible, and flow with life. Perfectionists, however, do not know how. They are not even able to relax. They have no awareness that they are already perfect and loving. Unable to trust (Erikson's first stage in the developmental cycle), such agers fear the unknown, a fear relentlessly denied. These toxic-prone, perfectionist, older adults refuse to admit that they no longer are able to contain their environment just to feel safe or restrain those inner compulsions. To be vulnerable is just too frightening, so they attack and lash out, the only control method they understand.

Relying on the ego's advice, toxic Ones become masters of the defense mechanism's projection and reaction formation. Placing their fears, faults, and imperfections onto others does give momentary relief, but to shift to the major task of Healthy agers in finding and embracing their whole Self and surrendering to a higher power seems almost unattainable.

Eventually, toxic agers may have a sense of guilt over what they have done, but their defenses prevent them from realizing, or admitting, the impact of their behavior on others. They only see themselves as Victims. Their constant complaining and passive-aggressive manipulations are now justified, and the toxic loop continues.

Enneagram Type Two. A different phenomenon occurs with the Two Helper, whose preferential strokes and energy come from helping others, a welcome attribute in our society. A word of warning, however; like all points on the Enneagram, Helpers too have a dark side: their inability to get their own needs met or to nourish themselves without manipulating others into needing them. Their strokes come from helping others, and when this help is authentic, their service is done in love and is the Helper's gift to society. Like all spiritual gifts, however, when out of balance and distorted, they become a weakness, and the Helper slides into the Unhealthy Self. For Helpers, this means they are using others to meet their own "need to be needed."

One adult child whom I interviewed, a type Two recovering co-Victim, put it succinctly when she wrote,

> I must take care of my own needs. I always seem to be able to see another's needs more clearly than my own. I am finding an inner voice saying to me now, before you agree, or before you offer, is this what you really want or is there something on your own agenda that is more important to you?

Then she went on to say,

> I remember an excellent workshop I attended years ago in which the leader suggested that some people hesitate to take care of themselves because they are afraid of losing the love of those they have been caring for. Take note, world. You'll have to love me for who I am because I'm not going to be your caretaker anymore!

A heavy statement that sounds self-centered until we recognize that a Two personality type is saying it. When this same adult child changes the second word in her first sentence from "must" to "am," she will be well on the road back to balance and reclaiming her true essence. Trouble is, as said before, super caregivers are welcomed and reinforced in our society. We *use* them, until their very gift of love, their strength, becomes a demanding compulsion in them—and their undoing. Until Helpers take care of themselves, they do not really have true love to give.

This is demonstrated in the toxic ager–Helper relationship when Unhealthy Helpers (whether it be service providers, caregivers, or adult children) find that if their services are unwanted and they are unable to express their feelings and nurture themselves, they become hostile or vindictive. The help that was to have been genuine has turned into the TA game triangle (see chapter 10), and the Helper becomes the Rescuer, then the Persecutor, and finally the co-Victim. Once again we see the toxic loop, and the insidiousness of this unceasing cycle.

Rarely do these agers, their families, or sometimes even professionals know how to deal with these incessant games and emotional outbursts or understand what is happening. One thing is certain: buried, long-stored, negative emotions and innate energy will be destructively unleashed if not prevented or dealt with early. All personality types can be susceptible to toxicity whenever they succumb to their own lower, unhealthy levels and compulsions and alienate themselves from their deepest, true Selves. To get mired in the dark side of our humanness is as simple as taking the wrong path on the Enneagram map.

Jung's Personality Theory

In the early 1900s, psychotherapist Carl Jung's break with Freud underscored the impact differences in personalities have on relationships, decisions, and responses. Jung was perplexed as to why he, Freud, and Adler all responded so differently to the same clinical data on patients. Their disagreements prodded Jung's search for answers and helped stimulate the publication of *Psychological Types* in 1921.

In his search, Jung became intrigued with the dualistic nature of life and the concept of opposites as found in the dominant and the least preferred or inferior functions of his personality types and the introvert-extravert attributes. It was in this dualism that Jung discovered why he and Freud saw things so differently. Their preferred functions were completely opposite, as were their attributes. Freud was an extraverted, sensing, thinking, judging (ESTJ) type with thinking as his dominant function and feeling as his inferior function. Jung, on the other hand, was an introverted, intuitive, feeling, perceiving (INFP) type with intuition as his dominant function and sensing as his inferior function.

Freud and Jung perceived situations and people from totally opposite perspectives. Each responded according to his own point of view, neither understanding nor respecting the other's perception. Conflicts flared between the two men, as they do among parents and children of different personality preferences. When this type of conflict occurs, whether between professionals and clients or adult children and parents, it is not a sign of toxicity. It is only a sign of differences in innate personality types.

Jung's focus on the unconscious also pointed out that professionals and laypersons both need to recognize the power and control the unconscious has over humans, particularly the person we perceive ourselves to be and the one we become.

Looking at the Shadow

In his book, *Make Friends with Your Shadow: How to Accept and Use Positively the Negative Side of Your Personality* (1981), Miller refers to the "Law of Psychic Balance." According to this law, one end of the continuum is the persona, the impersonation or mask we show to the outside world or public. The opposite end of the continuum is the shadow, the deeply embedded inner world. It is the parts that are disowned, unrecognized, undeveloped, unacknowledged, or underdeveloped, the original givens. The shadow can be both positive and negative, but it is usually what we do not want it to be, the feared dark side. The shadow may be seen by the outside world but rarely by ourselves, for it is the primitive, unrefined, animalistic, instinctive collection of impulses and reactions that so shock and appall us that we keep the lid on it to control and hide it from both ourselves and, futilely, others.

Most of us are so skilled in repressing our shadow we conveniently forget it even exists, depending on the degree or amount of vengeance or sourness we are covering up. This is where the problem with toxic agers shows up. When that protective cover begins to wear, when the spots get thin or are exposed to light and controls are weakened, the intolerable parts slip out. Fearful and confused, the toxics' first defense is to automatically project what they do not like in themselves onto the nearest person who will accept it. The toxics, seeing their projection in the other person, then turn around and attack that person for exhibiting what the toxics hate in themselves, producing again the toxic loop.

Generally, fear is felt when the hidden side is uncovered. As denoted by Jung, Erikson (1986), and the Enneagram, the task of aging is to develop, balance, and integrate all parts of us, especially the polar opposites, and the shadow that has been disowned in order to become whole. The goal is to unify these parts by embracing the shadow until its power and disquieting control is diminished, and we learn to use its potent energy productively, a difficult task but not impossible if the effort is made and we are open to spiritual transformation.

The Inferior Function

As the least preferred function of Jung's personality theory, the Inferior Function is rarely used. As the gateway to the shadow, however, it is significant. This Function explains why toxic agers cannot recognize their toxicity. When the Function is locked into its toxic loop (see chapter 10) and unable to accept a jolt that is strong enough to interrupt the endless negative feedback, toxic agers will not identify with it or own it, let alone integrate the polarities of each function and negative parts of their shadow. Their depth of fear and fragmentation is so deep they usually cannot, and won't, make the effort to work through their anger, hurt, or terror if they sense they are losing control.

Are Internal Multiple Selves an Answer?

Space allows for only a brief mention of the concept of Multiple Selves, a fairly recent spin-off from the clinical DSM-IV (American Psychiatric Association, 1994) Multiple Personality Disorder (MPD). Although multiple selves are also formed from severe and emotionally disturbing early childhood experiences, there is no dissociation trance as with MPD. Instead, these selves are similar to Jung's archetypes that are within each of us and guide us from both a positive and a negative perspective without our awareness, unless consciously evolved and used.

Some of these Selves, called "Multiple Realities" by Roberts (1992), are necessary and practical, such as the Protector, the Healer, the Teacher, or the Nurturing Parent. Others, such as the Troublemaker, the Toxic, the Inner Wounded Child, or the Violent, can be destructive, even evil. If not owned and left unattended and untamed with no limits and boundaries, these Selves can present themselves when least expected, spontaneously controlling in either a negative or a positive way. For toxic agers this means they could call on their internal Nurturing Parent for validation and comfort.

Is There a Biological Base for Toxicity?

It can be said that biology, the body, and the immune system are usually considered as part of Nature. What, then, is the connection with toxicity? Could neurobiology offer an explanation as to why toxic agers have so much trouble changing? Is toxicity inherited, learned, or a block?

I raise these questions only to stir thinking and to explore the premise that some emotional problems could be neurobiologically based. One example of a Nature-based possibility is the research of Candace Pert (1997), mentioned in an interview with Deepak Chopra (1997) regarding Pert's book, *Molecules in Emotions.*

According to Pert, neuropeptides (endorphins) and their receptors are the biochemical messengers of emotion that, through cellular signals, link the major autonomic systems and "translate information into physical reality," thus "literally transforming mind into matter" (Chopra, 1997, p. 3). This means that there is an internal connection between what Nature produces and the emotional impact on the body, stimulating the need for further exploration in the next two chapters.

Summary

Disagreeing with life-span developmentalists, typology theorists would say that personality type is innate and therefore could be considered a cause of toxic tendencies. Included also are definitions of toxicity that provide a common frame of reference; parts of four personality theories; other possible causes of toxicity identified with the concept of internal Multiple Selves; and the research on neuropeptides and their receptors, the emotional chemicals (mostly endorphins) that regulate moods and responses.

Gerontological theories appeared as early as the 1960s, when personality type was considered a key factor in understanding the different patterns of aging. Two particular studies classified the personality types, one of which was the classic Kansas City study of Neugarten et al. (1968).

The Enneagram also gives us some clues relative to the inherent personality tendencies that might cause toxicity. The essence of the Enneagram system, its symbol, structure, and unhealthy levels of the nine different personality types are described, including the two types most closely identified with toxic agers and their co-Victims, and the paths of movement each type takes toward well-being or toxicity.

Jung's personality theory is briefly examined, explaining the differences in individuals, the impact of the unconscious and the shadow, and the identification of polarized personality functions that offer some insights into excessive behavioral patterns.

Multiple Selves is a concept to be examined further because it presupposes that within each person are both negative and positive other Selves. Could one of these Selves be toxic?

Also presented for further study is the possible connection between neurobiology and toxicity as related to the emotional chemicals called neuropeptides, which are the information translators that unite the body and the mind.

Chapter 9

Is Nurture the Cause of Toxicity?

Is it possible that early environmental conditioning is the cause of toxicity in aging?

As stated in the last chapter, life-span developmentalists would argue that significant early influences in the environment shape and form the personality's lasting behavior. In that respect, environment would cause natural tendencies to be repressed and denied. To address this issue, several theories and models will be presented, including Jung, Erikson, Feil, the Recovery Movement, and Pert's research on the influence of emotions.

Conditioning

During our childhood, few of us would question whether the attitudes, beliefs, and values we were indoctrinated with fit our concept of who we are (Greenwald, 1977). Instead, that very conditioning becomes our self-concept and can hold us captive.

If parts of us are objectionable in the particular environment we are in, it is smart and comfortable to hide and disown them. The other parts are then adapted into a personality that fits that environment and the perceived image. We may not be true to our *Self*, but we are safe.

In support of this premise, Jung would say that the personality is developed or deformed by life experiences and modeling. For instance, he noticed that most children are quick to detect which behaviors are acceptable in their family and which are not. If independent thinking and free expression are punished by the parents and docility, sweetness, and unquestioning obedience bring favors, it is the acceptable behavior that is adopted by most children in order to survive. The individual's true self or true essence is denied and repressed, whereas the personality, the part that performs for others, develops. A self-illusion is formed, and a *life script* (TA) is unconsciously written.

Over time, the distorted self-perception, called the personality, is habituated, and the individual presumes that that image is the person they really are. Unfortunately, the unrecognized or disowned parts of us (which Jung named the shadow) are also who we are. Fearful of these parts, we push them into the unconscious, where they are hidden from view, only to erupt when our controls are weakened.

The Golden Shadow

Not all shadows, however, are negative. In keeping with Jung's concept of balance, there is a positive side, or golden shadow (Miller, 1989), that is also suppressed if unacceptable to the environment. It is often a talent or innate gift that was not allowed to flourish. Aptitudes and potentials, especially in toxic agers, are thus hidden deep within. Unless brought to light and embraced by both the self and others, these aptitudes remain undeveloped.

Environmental Impact

Few toxic agers are raised in an environment that is loving, open, caring, and accepting. It is not firmly structured with reason and boundaries within which there is the freedom for curiosity, risk taking, and expression of feelings. Toxics are more likely to be raised in an environment that is abusive, either verbally, physically, emotionally, or sexually. It is also demanding, rigid, suppressive, and full of "shoulds," "oughts," and "threats." Freedom to grow, experiment, or express natural feelings is nonexistent.

When the feelings of emotionally abused children are denied expression, it is only a matter of time before these children lose touch with their feelings, ultimately finding it impossible to manifest them appropriately and responsibly. Instead, the feelings are suppressed and buried deep in the unconscious, usually as the shadow, only to rise up in old age as untamed, disruptive patterns and unfinished business.

Erikson's Life-Cycle Stages

In his eight stages of the life-cycle, Erikson distinguishes between the ideal developmental adaptation and the maladaption of individuals to their environment as they progress through the different levels. While in his 80's, Erikson expanded this focus to the reintegration of these stages and the reversing of the process as aging occurs. An example is presented in his last book, written in collaboration with his wife and Helen Kivnick:

> [It is the task of those in the last period of life to] bring into balance the tension between a sense of integrity, of enduring comprehensiveness, and an opposing sense of despair, of dread and hopelessness. (1986, p. 54)

The Eriksons charged older adults to develop integrity; to integrate and form an enduring balance of their opposite feelings, tensions, and subparts in order to become unified and whole; to accept and embrace the parts of themselves that are offensive and unlovable; and to unite all the elements of their *beingness*. These offensive elements are what Jung called the "shadow"; the parts of our psyche* that have gone unrecognized and whose ownership must be claimed before wholeness and the wisdom of Erikson's eighth stage of integrity rather than despair can be experienced.

Integrating the integrity stage, however, is only part of the process. Agers are asked to go back through each of the seven other psychosocial stages and reintegrate or reincorporate the earlier stage themes into new ways of living appropriate to their age. This means they need to undertake anew the struggle to reconcile, retravel, reexperience, and come to terms with the tensions of all of Erikson's stages and their maladaptations by balancing them first in descending order, then back up again in ascending order. Admittedly, this is a difficult journey and may be impossible for most toxic agers, who seem to be stuck at the first stage of development: trust.

With blockage at trust (Table 9.1) and the ascension process subsequently incomplete, the likelihood of toxic agers completing Erikson's descension process is remote. Instead, underdeveloped or distorted perceptions and responses will continue because more evolved stages will also be psychologically contaminated.

If movement through the stages is interfered with by environmental forces, maladaptive or noxious behavior and tendencies of withdrawal, compulsiveness, ruthlessness, rejection, disdain, shamelessness, maladjustment, and overextension (Erikson et al.,

TABLE 9.1 Erikson's Eight Life-Cycle Stages of Development

Ideal		Maladaptions
Integrity	and	Despair
Generativity	and	Stagnation
Intimacy	and	Isolation
Identity Cohesion	and	Role Confusion
Industriousness	and	Inferiority
Initiative	and	Guilt
Autonomy	and	Shame/Doubt
Trust	and	Mistrust

Note. Themes are reversed to show the reintegration process. Adapted from *Vital Involvement in Old Age: The Experience of Old Age in Our Time* (p. 45), by E. H. Erikson, J. M. Erikson, and H. Q. Kivnick, 1986, New York: Norton & Company.

1986, p. 45) will emerge, symptomatic of many toxic, or emotionally abused agers.

As time passes, it is common for people with these maladaptive tendencies to transform them into negative coping skills and defense mechanisms simply to survive. Eventually this behavior evolves into habitually ingrained, unconscious, destructive patterns, the norm for toxic agers.

The Feil Method and Life Task Theory

Naomi Feil, geriatric social worker, began working with mal-oriented people in 1963, and by 1980 had developed her theory of Validation: The Feil Method. Early exposure to the old in her parents' home for the care of the elderly stimulated Feil's interest in the old, an interest later enhanced by specialized training and years of professional practice with the agitated and mal-oriented old-old.

Early in her extensive training, Feil was impressed with Erikson's theory of Life-Cycle Stages, later adapting and expanding it to form a framework for her own theory and work. Her methods and principles regarding the mal-oriented are best depicted in the instructional video, "Myrna, The Mal-oriented" (1997). Geared to professional and nonprofessional caregivers, the video teaches how to empathize and validate the very old afflicted with both aggressive Alzheimer-like behavior and toxicity.

In her Life Task Chart (Table 9.2), Feil drops two of Erikson's stages, calls her stages "tasks," and adds the task of *Resolution versus Vegetation*, plus the results of failing to achieve each task. To Feil the Resolution task is the most critical in the aging process, particularly if the sixth task, or Erikson's Integrity Stage of Wisdom, is not attained by the time the old-old phase of aging is reached. Maladaptation often sets in, and progresses into Malorientation if tasks are left unfinished, and conflicts unresolved.

Both Feil and Erikson emphasize that if older adults fail to do the developmental work of aging and do not achieve each of the

TABLE 9.2 Feil's Life Task Chart

Developmental level	Task	Failure-to-achieve task
1. Infancy	Learn to Trust when frustrated	Dis-Trust "I'm Unlovable."
2. Childhood	Learn to control bowel functions. Follow rules	Shame. Guilt. Blame. "I always mess up."
3. Adolescent	Find own identity. Rebel. Separate from parental authority.	Insecurity. Role-diffusion. "I'm only somebody if I'm loved."
4. Adult	Intimacy. Share raw feelings. Responsible for feelings, failures, and successes.	Isolation Dependency
5. Mid-years	Generate new activity when old roles wear out. Retire to something new.	Stagnation. Holding-on to outworn roles.
6. Old Age	Tie-up living. Find inner strength. Integrity. Blend the past with the present. Set new goals.	Despair "I might as well be dead."
7. Old-Old Age	Resolution of the past.	Vegetation

Note. Adaptation of Erickson's Life-Cycle Stages. From VIF *Validation®: The Feil Method—How to Help Disoriented Old-Old* (p. 21), by N. Feil, 1992, Cleveland: Feil Productions. Copyright 1992 by Naomi Feil. Reprinted with author's permission.

tasks at the stage for which it was designed, maladaptive behavior can be expected. Inner turmoil and distress are the by-products.

Descriptive Expectations

Although not usually identified, toxic emotional abusers often feel imprisoned by their own fears, guilt, anger, and hurt if these are not owned, dealt with, or integrated—both internally and externally—at early developmental stages. According to Feil, painful, stored feelings may appear to the very old in a *disguised* form as memories of those earlier feelings are triggered. Inappropriate behavior then erupts from the agers involved, disturbing everyone around, including the agers themselves, who often do not understand what is happening and struggle excessively to maintain rigid control of old perceptions and self-images.

Because toxic agers rarely achieve Integrity, they do not know how to responsibly manage environmental forces, or even believe they have the power to choose a different course. Erikson would classify them as maladaptive. To Feil they would be mal-oriented, a category that represents the first of the three stages of her Disorientation Theory. In that theory, maladaption is the preliminary behavior that leads to mal-orientation, which leads to disorientation, which leads to institutionalization. This implies a possible disturbing progression as the description of Feil's mal-oriented stage amazingly parallels my description of what I would call the more advanced stage of toxicity in agers, with maladaptation being the early stage.

According to Feil, the mal-oriented old and old-old are unhappy frustrated people, better known as whiners and blamers. They apparently do not know how to get their act together, adapt to life, cope, work through their dysfunctions, or love and validate themselves. The reason? Mal-oriented never learned to trust, to complete that first stage and task of development. The possibility that they could learn to trust, or to love later in life, never occurs to them. Instead they reinforce their ego and dissipate their pain by blaming others for their problems. Feelings are repressed and then projected onto unsuspecting family members, caregivers, or friends, especially the unacknowledged anger, a cover for fear and hurt.

Theories do make it easier to understand the steps of dysfunction. For example, moving down her chart, Feil theorizes that distrust leads to unlovableness, lack of control leads to blame, lack of identity leads to insecurity and role confusion, lack of intimacy leads to isolation and dependency, lack of new activity leads to stagnation, and lack of integrity leads to despair. The progression leads to a sense of foreboding. Then it follows that if there is no Resolution, there is Vegetation.

The Recovery Movement

Pervasive throughout the text has been the implication that emotionally damaging experiences in the early childhood environment are correlated to toxicity. Therefore, it is not surprising that I have chosen to include the Recovery Movement and its inner child emphasis to toxic agers.

Two books of the Recovery Movement are pertinent to the toxicity syndrome because they offer clues as to the possible cause of toxicity when good intentions in parenting, carried to an extreme, also become destructive.

In her book *The Emotional Incest Syndrome: What to Do When a Parent's Love Rules Your Life* (1990), Pat Love, marriage and family therapist, suggests that emotional incest is a form of role reversal or style of parenting in which the child becomes the parent's source of emotional support. The child is trained to suppress his or her own needs and identity in order to meet the needs of the parents, to please them and make them happy (a type Two, Unhealthy Enneagram personality type). Rarely is either the parent or the child aware of what is really happening. Both are so tied up emotionally that parent–child boundaries are fuzzy or lost, although they may look ideal to the outsider. The problem is, these children eventually lose the sense of who they really are and have no idea how to identify their needs or use the energy of a deepening, concealed anger to correct the situation later in life.

Toxic agers, like these children, are usually taught to suppress their feelings and thoughts, keep their mouths shut, do what they are told, and work hard. Emotions like hurt and anger are buried. Missing also is a model of how to truly love, both themselves and others. Survival is based on pleasing parents and unquestioning obedience. Coping requires controlling and hiding their own feelings.

In *For Your Own Good: Hidden Cruelty in Child-rearing and the Roots of Violence*, Alice Miller used different terms, but it is the same message. Published in the United States in 1990, this book stirred the educational and psychoanalytical worlds. For some, its provocative pronouncements jolted conditioned norms or, as Gurdjieff would say, shook the system.

After 20 years as a psychoanalyst, Miller has renounced the theory and practice of psychoanalysis as it is related to child abuse. Hillman and Ventura (June, 1992) feel that psychoanalysis tends to leave the abused stuck in the emotions of a traumatized memory and sets up a victim mentality. Caroline Myss calls it *woundology* in her latest book, *Why People Don't Heal and How They Can* (1997). Miller sees the abused *cemented* in the confusions of their childhood. They remain, like toxics, victims. Neither knows how to find solutions. They have not yet learned, as depicted in so many biographies and art, how buried resentment, bitterness, and feelings of worthlessness can be a depressant to productive growth.

Miller goes even further. Believing (like Hillman) that the focus should be on the developmental process, the causes, and the consequences of the wounding and not on the symptoms or the act itself, Miller has labeled her theory "Poisonous Pedagogy" (Miller, 1990).

"We can protect ourselves from poison only if it is clearly labeled as such" (Miller, 1990, p. vii). Poison is not recognized if it is camouflaged in the harsh, commanding words, "do as you're told, don't ask questions, it's for your own good."

Pedagogy is "the art of teaching" and can be effective or harmful, developmental or crippling. Regardless of value, when pedagogy is called parenting, it is rarely questioned. For Miller, harmful parenting under the guise of "training" is only the transfer of cruelty.

Some parents use this type of training to consciously delude themselves into believing they are teaching their child to be "good." It is a training that may even be praised by society because it molds children into "perfect" sons or daughters and "ideal" citizens. It is a training that models the use of projected displacement and starts when the child is very young, at a time when there is little questioning or awareness of what is actually going on. It is an upbringing that accelerates the Enneagram One personality type and its toxic-prone Unhealthy Level. Few outsiders notice what is going on, but the children know. It is modeling that teaches them how to avoid feeling, independent thinking, problem solving, and self-worth: the seeds of toxicity.

Training of this kind, in the form of disguised conditioning and manipulation, is usually received and understood by children to be for their own good. This was evidenced in my interviews in the way the toxic agers responded to my questions: "How did your parents relate to each other? Did you feel their love?"

The nonverbals and pained pauses were descriptively clear, but the common words were "Well, they worked so hard to provide. They were strict, but they wanted me to be good. They wanted me to be strong."

Only one interviewee broke the accepted pattern. She responded with the following:

INTERVIEWEE: I never saw them kiss each other. They didn't show any affection . . . nor toward me either.

DAVENPORT: How did you feel about that?

INTERVIEWEE: Angry! (Then a little laugh slipped out.)

DAVENPORT: Did you ever ask them for any love?

INTERVIEWEE: I didn't realize until I was older that other people were doing that. I never felt close to my mother . . . nor to my father. Sometimes I really hated him.

A sudden surprised look then broke the silence.

INTERVIEWEE: I'm being very honest. I don't tell very many people that.

The Indoctrination

As part of pedagogical indoctrination, any problem that arises is the child's fault, not the parents'. The teaching is usually through threats, fear, punishment, and humiliation or through seductive and enticing manipulation, feigned friendliness or illness, or other subtle devices. Both approaches compel the child to forgo—literally give up—his or her own feelings, thinking, sensing, and natural inclinations in order to conform. The child unknowingly chooses to make the parents' teachings his or her own reality. In order to survive, emotions are cut off; the pain then disappears. What the child does not know, however, is that these buried feelings may erupt later, often in old age, as untamed, unrecognized, animalistic outbursts.

An additional problem for children raised under "poisonous pedagogy" is that they are taught to lie, a pattern that repeats itself. Even at 55, adult children of toxic parents find it simpler to lie to a toxic parent than to be honest. How better to cover up feelings and thoughts? The smile, when you're feeling hateful? The promise of a call or visit never intended? Then the example of negative coping modeled for the grandchildren?

Rewards are also part of the "poisonous pedagogy" conditioning but only if the child shows self-control and prompt obedience and is strong. For the child, desperate for positive strokes, these rewards are significant. Negative rewards, such as the withholding of validations, restrictions, silence, and withdrawal, as well as harsh physical punishment for normal crying, reacting spontaneously, speaking before thinking, being impatient, interrupting, or displaying any autonomous childhood behavior or independent thinking, however, are more common.

Children of this type of parenting have one function: to meet the needs of the parent. Fear and dependency are the result. As with Love's emotional incest syndrome, this form of dependency continues throughout adulthood and old age unless the perceptual feedback loop is shocked and the toxics awaken to their addiction. If there is no awakening, the entire syndrome will be repeated, again and again, in the next generation when the abused are now free to unconsciously dump their pent-up, forbidden, and repressed anger and rage on their children or spouses—to become the abuser.

For the 50- to 65-year-old care providers, however, who are now better acquainted with their parents than they ever wanted to be, it becomes more and more difficult. They soon feel torn between a justified inner rage and an early conditioning that says, Thou shalt love, honor, and obey thy parents. Thou shalt suppress thine own emotions; sacrifice to make them happy. After all, look at all they have done for you! Don't be an ungrateful child. Loyalty is primary, and so is silence. Don't seek outside support.

Parental Ignorance?

Maybe it is possible that toxic parents do not understand that emotional needs are as important as food, clothing, shelter, limits, and control. Maybe it is possible that they do not understand how discipline via shame and criticism becomes emotionally damaging and that children need to be consistently affirmed, loved, and valued, meaning daily hugs, touch, and listening, in an environment of trust that says, "I'll be there for you—always." Maybe it is possible that some parents do not know that children need to be taught how to nourish and love themselves in order to build and maintain a sense of worth.

Does this ignorance have to mean that the unresolved fears assimilated by toxic agers as children from verbal, emotional, and physically abusive parenting must now, because of diminishing self-controls, be displaced onto their own adult children and anyone else within reach, causing more toxicity? Does it mean that the cause of toxicity is an assumption that toxics never learned *how* to love and nourish themselves or effectively cope with their environment? Does it mean that toxicity could be connected to internal cellular responses to perceived external messages from environmental stimuli?

The Internal Environment

When most of us think of environment, we think of the forces outside of ourselves, the external. I want to shift that thinking and expand my questions on neurobiology from chapter 8 to another possibility, an internal environment inside our body. In a follow-up of Pert's research (Chopra, 1997), I am proposing that within us is a biologic environment in which the cells and major systems of the body are in constant communication and are affected and change according to the messages they receive from the interlinking network of emotional chemicals or information carriers known as neuropeptides. If the messages transmitted, processed, and stored are negative, as with toxicity, it would seem that the body would respond with a breakdown in the immune system, causing a blockage of endorphin releases and thus materializing into negative moods and behavior?

According to Pert, if the body network is overloaded with "suppressed trauma or undigested emotions," the peptides are prevented from flowing freely. This collapses the autonomic systems that the peptides regulate down to a simple feedback loop, disrupting the normal healing process (Chopra, September 1997, p. 8). Subsequently, we can speculate that if the emotions of fear and anger are suppressed, the immune cell receptors are affected and the autonomic limbic system is blocked, causing nature's normal healing response to be weakened and lead to "dis-ease."* In essence, the mind becomes matter and psychosomatic illness follows.

An example of this can be viewed in the developmental story of T's early life. The older college student, and my counselee, was first mentioned in chapter 6 in the description of the impact of a toxic ager on a college.

T's story (as she told it to me) began when her father walked out on her mother the night T was born, loudly proclaiming that T was not his child. This departure started a pattern of threats and his leaving the family several times during T's childhood. When she was a toddler, her father was gone for 2 years. Finally, in desperation, T's mother took her 2-year-old and traveled 2,000 miles to beg him to come home. She was convinced she could never make it on her own. Even his terrible temper tantrums, alcoholism, job instabilities, periods of unemployment, and beatings did not offset her debilitating fear of abandonment. It was a fear that hung over the family like a dark cloud. For years, T had disdainfully watched her mother go after her father and bring him back, always for more suffering. Then one day as a teenager, T could stand it no longer. She physically stood in the doorway to block her mother from again following her father. It did not work. T's mother had settled for the Victim role.

During T's preschool years she was confined to the house and not allowed to play with the other children in the low-income area where they lived. With no siblings or other children to socialize with, T learned few interactive social skills.

As T grew older, her father (when he was present) would occasionally, and impulsively, decide to help her with her lessons. T proclaimed,

It was a disaster. Whenever I asked him to clarify something, he became annoyed and impatient, called me stupid, and would scream at me saying,

"You never can do anything right." One time it got so bad, he almost strangled me.

In junior and senior high school, the students, according to T, would scorn her, call her names, go through her personal things, destroy her projects, and

accuse me of everything. The teachers and administration didn't help either. They just talked about me in staff meetings, so there was no point in complaining. I just put a different name on my papers so I could get a better grade.

In her preteens T was sexually molested by "some boys," which reinforced her fearful, defensive, almost paranoid, nature. As with her father, T commented that she learned quickly to stay out of the way. This meant giving up trying to date.

By college T was perfecting her ability to protect herself by controlling the environment and attacking before she was attacked. It usually worked. An example was the time one teacher started to criticize T's classwork. With a smirk on her face, T proudly announced, "I verbally let him have it."

Later, after several years in a community college, T experienced what she called "her biggest blow." She got sick and was forced to drop out of school, a place where she had finally begun to feel like someone. She could get good grades and that meant a few positive strokes.

T's illness was a general malaise, including dysentery and depression. It lasted 10 years. No one believed she was actually ill. Because of sporadic attendance, T had been given a choice: be in your classes or drop. She put herself in therapy, only to be accused of "enjoying her illness." Upset and frustrated, T felt her only choice was to return home and live with her unstable mother. Her father was now gone for good. Troubled and depressed, T confined herself to the house for 5 years.

T was not aware that her lack of self-nourishment and perceived rejections, together with the bitterness and anger that had been suppressed and held in for so many years, would eventually, as postulated by Pert (1997), accumulate in her body cells and convert to a chemical toxin. Neither did she realize that projecting them onto others could, as Steinbeck wrote in 1962, "kill the soul" and make both her and her scapegoats co-Victims. She also was not conscious that her persistent identification with her childhood wounds and environmental dysfunctions left her addicted to her past, and (as Myss would say), stuck in her own *woundology* (Myss, 1997) and self-pity.

Once T opened up, every conversation reverted to her "broken record-like" tales of woe. They were experiences that justified her attitude and behavior (and unrecognized toxicity); legitimized her "right to be manipulative, bitter, or angry" (Myss, 1997, p. 20); and facilitated her need for a sense of control and power in order to feel safe.

Unfortunately, by keeping self-destructive perceptions alive in her memory cells, much of T's life force energy was dissipated. Unable, or unwilling, to nourish herself, she used others (like suckers) to resupply her energy drain; a tactic that also supported her Victim consciousness and toxic games. Now T's woundology was her identity and the only way she knew to relate to others.

Summary

Life-span developmentalists will assert that the environment shapes and molds the personality's lasting behavior. Early conditioning and indoctrination will hold the individual captive if a negative response pattern and self-concept are habituated. Any personal attributes, both positive and negative, that are not acceptable to influential environmental forces (such as significant others) are suppressed and disowned, becoming the shadow. As stated by Jung, the personality is either developed or deformed by life experiences.

Erikson, in his Life-Cycle Stages, theorizes that individuals develop in stages and that failure to complete the early stages causes maladaptation in future stages. This is evidenced by toxic agers, who are often stuck in the first stage, having learned early not to trust their environment to protect and care for them. These agers are predictably incapable of reversing the stages of development, as proposed by Erikson, and of "reintegrating" all eight stages in order to fulfill the process of successful aging.

Feil, in her Life Task Theory, further expands on Erikson's Stages and emphasizes not only the development of Integrity but also the task of Resolution, which enables agers to avoid imprisonment in their own fears, guilt, and anger and the advancement to maladaptation and malorientation.

The Recovery Movement stresses the importance of effective, early childhood training and nurturance and that inner wounding occurs when the teaching or modeling is dysfunctional. This is vividly depicted in Love's "Emotional Incest Syndrome" and Miller's "Poisonous Pedagogy" theories.

Pert's cutting edge, neurobiological research with receptors and neuropeptides (called chemical emotions) as regulators of autonomic systems implies that the internal environment is also a factor in how the body's cellular network system interacts and responds to emotions, where the mind and body become one and can produce the chronic psychosomatic responses so common among toxic agers.

An example of Pert's theory and Myss's concept of woundology is portrayed in the early history of T, the 76-year-old, toxic college student referred to in chapter 6 as an illustration of the impact of toxicity on higher education.

Chapter 10

Is It Nature and Nurture?

It is not Nature. It is not Nurture. It is both.

It is the daily task of maintaining a balance between innate givens and developmental environmental forces. It is the interaction between the conscious and the unconscious, reality and illusion, free thinking and conditioning, and the mind and the body—until they become one.

It was Carl Jung who identified early that when people fight against the outer world, they are also battling something similar within themselves.

It is this battle, the inner conflict in toxic agers between who they are and what they perceive they should be that creates much of their inner turmoil, misdirected behavior, and neurosis. Their environment did not teach them to balance their inner and outer forces or to develop and maintain a stable, self-loving response pattern. Nevertheless, that is no excuse for toxic agers to negate their responsibility for learning it on their own.

Personal Responsibility. According to the theories described in chapter 8, we are born with certain personality traits and tendencies. The development of that personality and its true characteristics, however, depends to a great extent on how each of us chooses to interpret and respond to the signals and messages received from our early childhood environment, especially if that environment is nurturing and enhances our true essence or tends to suppress its development.

Transactional Analysis

Transactional analysis (TA), a behavioral psychology developed by Eric Berne in the 1950s and popularized by Tom Harris in his book *I'm OK, You're Not OK* (1967), demonstrates some of the interactive dynamics between individual choice and environmental impact.

Life Scripts

Claude Steiner, a student of Eric Berne's and original Research Director of Berne's San Francisco Social Psychiatry Seminars, developed Berne's initial thinking on life scripts, a concept significant to the Victim consciousness of toxic agers. The term "script" comes from the idea of a theater production. It is the blueprint from which individuals build their identity, where they develop the plot, staging, scenery, characters, props, and drama for the rest of their lives. It is a personal play, written when each person is a child between the ages of 2 and 6. The shape and form of the script depends on the child's instinctive perceptions and decisions regarding the meaning of verbal and nonverbal messages received from significant others in his or her life, usually parents.

Unfortunately, these scripts are engraved in the minds of children consistent with how they interpret those early environmental messages, not on actual reality, and are played out accordingly. Verification of the events that led to these interpretations are rare; therefore, it is somewhat frightening to discover that there is no way of knowing if the interpretations are accurate. They may be an illusion, unconsciously designed to fit a self-ascribed image that subsequently unfolds into a negative drama. To ensure a continuance of the script, it is recorded and stored on a mental *tape*, then replayed over and over unless a conscious choice is made to finally stop. It is only then that old environmental interpretations no longer dictate daily behavior. Victimization is then finally disrupted.

Hillman Reinforcement

This thinking was reinforced by psychoanalyst James Hillman when he accused the Recovery Movement of turning America into a victim mentality (Hillman & Ventura, 1992) by emphasizing the "wounded child" and encouraging people to dredge up memories that he felt excused behavior and discouraged self-responsibility. Even if these memories were fictionalized, they represented ego illusions that governed perceptions and subsequent behavioral responses, thus explaining why toxic agers make themselves into psychological Victims.

Hillman does not deny that traumas occur. What is more important, he says, is *how* we remember them. It is not the actual experience that is so critical but what is done with the emotions and awakened memories.

Toxic agers are more inclined to rehash and lament over their memories (as shown by the case of T), than work through the pain. Awareness is not friendly. Even if these emotional abusers are aware and choose to face their emptiness, their needs, and their longing for love and attachment, can they make the difficult transformational journey? Would they even want to undertake the task if they are determined to keep the dark shadow side and the compulsions under controlled denial? That would only reinforce the belief that they are not strong and no longer in control.

Changing the Script

According to TA, since the original scripts were written when we were children, it is possible to rewrite them as adults. Each of us has the power to change a negative and toxic script into a positive one; that is, if we want to. The major drawback is that we may, unconsciously, sabotage our own good intentions and effort. Early decisions are often intuitively creative because they help to protect, defend, and maintain the ego personality at the time. Over the years, however, our true essence is usually blocked when habituated behavior is no longer beneficial.

Change is not easy. As understood in TA theory, old tapes cannot be erased, but they can be written over, modified, and revised, changing the script. This means we are in charge, and it *is* our responsibility to reclaim, restore, and accept who we are, shadow and all. It is our responsibility to integrate, as Erikson and Feil say, all the life-cycle stages. When we do, wholeness is possible. Illusions, negative scripts, game *payoffs*, and others to blame are no longer needed. The choices are ours.

Stroking

Berne based his theory of stroking on Spitz's (1945) study in the early 1940s of hospitalized infants deprived of handling over long periods of time. Spitz discovered that without regular touching and cuddling, these babies would sink into irreversible decline and succumb to disease. He called it *emotional deprivation* (Spitz, 1945).

Relating these findings to his psychiatric patients, Berne claimed that a cure for emotional deprivation was positive stroking, or units of recognition. Negative stroking was the cause of disease and included not only neglect but also all forms of verbal and emotional abuse. To Berne, strokes were a way of furthering either the positive or the negative life script.

This is further seen in Bowlby's series on Attachment and Loss Theory (1967–1980). If the positive strokes of unconditional love that induce trust and security are missing in early life, attachment is inhibited. According to Sue Johnson in her article "The Biology of Love" (1997, p. 38), Bowlby stated that the need to love and be loved by an irreplaceable other is innate. If the intimate bonding of this attachment does not occur and there is no responsive, reliable, and trusting connection, a neurophysiological response may subsequently create cruel behavior in adults (Johnson, 1997, p. 39).

In TA terms, the early stage of this kind of cruel behavior may occur when toxic agers reject the very positive strokes that could affirm and validate them; strokes such as compliments, support, nonjudgmental listening, and caring. Instead, by refusing positive strokes, agers promote and uphold their "Not OK" script.

It takes years, but in time toxic agers unconsciously build an impenetrable wall (the personality armor mentioned in the section on gerontology theories) that hides their pain and reinforces the negative self-image and script so cleverly designed to protect them as children. To maintain this script and Victim self-perception, however, these agers must now give, and provoke, negative strokes just to feel alive. Some of these are depicted by the nonverbal scowls, the sighs of disgust and martyrdom, the silent treatment, or the seductive verbal putdowns, such as Can't you ever do anything right?, You don't love me anymore, How could you be so mean?, and You just want me to die. With these invectives, and worse, toxics continue to prove to themselves that the world they see and experience is out to get them. They are the victims. They sense no responsibility for setting up this kind of environment or its feedback.

Ego States

Designated by Berne as personality subparts, *ego states* are usually pictured as three circles stacked on top of each other representing the Parent, Adult, and Child within each of us (Figure 10.1). Each state can be readily identified by its specific characteristics. The Parent ego state possesses the values, traditions, customs, conscience, and shoulds and oughts that control our behavior, keeping us in line. The Adult ego state is computer-like, with no feelings. It is the objective part, the data collector, problem solver, and rational reasoner. The Child has the emotions and the energy, is spontaneous, and acts with no conscience or logic, only feelings.

Two of the ego states are subdivided. The Parent, for example, has two parts: the Nurturing Parent and the Critical or Controlling Parent. The Child ego state has three parts: the Adaptive Child, the Little Professor, and the Natural or Rebel Child (James & Jongeward, 1973).

All of the subdivided parts (pictured by the dotted lines in Figure 10.1) have both a positive and a negative side, the key being to keep the sides balanced. If unbalanced on the negative side, the Critical Parent will criticize and discount everything and everyone with which it comes in contact. If the sides are in balance,

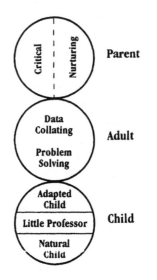

FIGURE 10.1 Ego states.

however, the positive side is free to make sound judgments and assessments of situations, behavior, and systems based not on fear and projected distortions but on values, laws, and the loving thing to do.

The ego state subparts most relevant to toxic agers are the Critical Parent and the Little Professor (Figure 10.2). In the toxic ager, the negative part of the Critical Parent consumes the positive part, leaving the controlling Critical Parent dogmatic and dominant. The Adult ego state is minimally functional, and the negative, manipulative side of the Little Professor is out of control. Although these are clever survival tactics, invaluable in times of distress, they become destructive when clung to and used inappropriately. In addition, because the Child ego state has no conscience or thoughts of future consequences, it can get into endless trouble if left to operate by itself with no firm, Nurturing Parent ego state to keep it under control or Adult ego state to provide some facts and problem-solving strategies. Because both the Adult

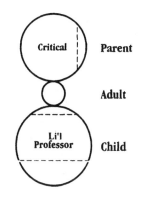

FIGURE 10.2   Substates.

and the Nurturing Parent in the toxic ager are almost nonfunc-
tioning, the toxic ager is prone to overuse all parts of the negative
Child ego state, especially the manipulative Little Professor.

In emotionally healthy, successful agers, all three ego states
are in balance. They work together as a team toward becoming
integrated and whole. The Adult ego state acts as the executor,
or monitor, between the other two states, enabling all to function
as an effective, harmonious unit. With the toxic ager, however,
the ego states are out of balance. The negative substates of the
Child ego state and the Critical Parent are the ones in control,
possessed by unresolved emotional tensions, conflicts, and pain
from the past. All interact with and influence their environment,
as well as being the ones most likely to play games.

Psychological Games

As noted in previous chapters, toxic agers and their co-Victims
are skilled game players. Berne's games are not the activity games
that children play but are transactions based on deep psychological premises that are out of the awareness of the Adult ego state
and the Nurturing Parent. Consequently, these games are very
effective in maintaining and advancing negative behavior. These
games also serve a purpose for toxic agers by

- inhibiting honesty in relationships
- furthering a negative life script
- collecting negative strokes
- reinforcing being Not Ok
- producing a bad feeling payoff and
- preventing time for intimacy

Psychological games are not played with conscious awareness. They require at least two people "hooked" into each other, a significant point because it means there is always a co-Victim. Both must know the rules of the games that are then automatically executed and without thought. Games are repetitious, have a hidden agenda or ulterior motive, and continue as long as participants are willing to play and follow the unwritten rules. Players know when the game has ended because they are left with a "bad-feeling-payoff." This feeling may last for minutes, a few hours, or a few days until another player is found and the game is replayed.

Critical to game playing is the fact that the unconscious (possibly the shadow) is in control. Games can come from the Parent ego state, but the predominant role is carried by the emotional energy of the Child, especially the Little Professor. It is an energy that is so powerful it can overcome both the Parent and the Adult ego states if permitted to take charge. When this happens, problems quickly arise because the Child ego state operates without a conscience or any sense of future consequences. It becomes an unguided missile if the Nurturing Parent abdicates its role. Therefore, it is crucial that boundaries are set within which the Child is safe, loved, and free to develop, something often missing in a toxic's growth period.

Game Analysis

Since most games are played out of the Child and Parent ego states, it is helpful to visualize how they interact and keep the toxicity in agers active. In Figure 10.3, the arrows depict the conscious transactions, and the dotted lines show the unconscious, hidden agenda. Both transactions must occur at the same time to constitute a game. Because game playing is how members

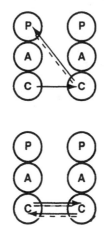

FIGURE 10.3   Game analysis.

of toxic families communicate, the Little Professor substate in each participant learns early how to creatively find ways to keep the games going. It means survival. Through conditioning, it takes only a certain look, word, or mannerism and the game is on. The Critical Parent knows exactly which buttons to push so the Child within is instantly hooked. Unfortunately, until brought into the unemotional Adult ego state and stopped, the toxic games go on infinitely as models for the next generations. Instead of stopping the toxicity, the other players in the toxic's environment are now maintaining and intensifying the games, deepening and holding the ager's power. Not aware of the interactive dynamics of games, the other players simply continue to feed the *toxic loop.*

Karpman's Triangle

It was Steve Karpman, a student of Berne, who first described the interactive dynamics of game playing, portraying it as an upside-down triangle (Figure 10.4). He identified three components of the game: the Persecutor, the Rescuer, and the Victim, with the Victim always found at the bottom point. Names were purposely capitalized to distinguish the players from true persecutors and legitimate rescuers and victims.

Perpetual movement is the dynamic of Game Theory because players frequently shift parts, playing all roles of the games, with one exception. Toxic agers play the Victim and Persecutor roles exclusively.

For example, in the familiar game "I'm Only Trying to Help," the toxic Victims immediately hook into the care providers who, despite good intentions, find themselves in the "Big R" Rescuer role. Within minutes these same Rescuers may discover they are behaving like Persecutors, then suddenly become Victims, unconsciously sucked into the interactive dynamics of the game. Some overcaring adult children and gerontology professionals are particularly susceptible to these seductive tactics.

Types of Games

After years of observing the dynamics of these games, Berne and his followers noticed that particular patterns began to appear. Based on these patterns, game types were identified and named. Most applicable to toxic agers and co-Victims are the following:

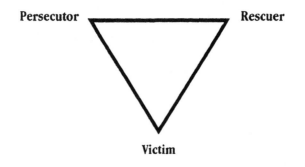

FIGURE 10.4   Karpman's Triangle.

- I'm Only Trying to Help! (see previous example)
- Poor Me
- Yes, But . . . Why Don't You? (the helper hook)
- Wooden Leg (I can't because of . . .)
- Look What I'm Doing For You . . .
- If Only . . .
- Do Me For (Do for me)
- If It Weren't For You . . . (I would have . . .)
- Lets You and Him Fight
- Uproar
- NIGYSOB or Gotcha

The list grows longer when games customized to fit specific players are included. The interaction of toxic interior emotions and enabling exterior environments causes continuous evolution of the toxicity.

Ego States and Games

Unfortunately, in my work with people who associate daily with toxic agers, especially adult children, I find few who are able to discern in which ego state the toxic ager is in order to achieve accurate direct and honest communication. Adult children mistakenly assume that just because their parents are adults, they are in their Adult ego state and can communicate rationally and objectively. This assumption is misleading and troublesome. Toxic agers do not function out of their Adult ego state. Consequently, most adult children, and some service providers, are hooked by the toxic ager's manipulative Little Professor. When caught, these care providers slide immediately, and unconsciously, into their own matching, negative Child ego state and one or more of the many game options available. Emotions and defenses run high, spewed words are regretted, and the game and toxicity accelerate.

Defense Mechanisms

Sigmund Freud's daughter and student, Anna, is credited with articulating and clarifying defense mechanisms. They are generally purported to be unconscious strategies that protect the self-image, or ego position, particularly when clinging to self-deceptions. Although self-defeating, defense mechanisms are a quick fix for momentarily easing ego bruises. These mechanisms temporarily protect the false self from emotional hurt and help maintain the ego images and self-illusions through the Cybernetic* system of a closed feedback loop.

Interestingly, Cybernetics (see the end of this chapter) presents a different perspective of defense mechanisms than normally assumed. In Cybernetic theory, defense mechanisms are *not* unconscious; they are just perceived to be such. They simply happen so fast no one is aware of any conscious thought process. This means that defense mechanisms are actually immature, learned strategies that are created by the brain and nervous system from the trial and error of early problem-solving days. As time passes, they become habituated "servo-mechanisms" (Maltz, 1969) that respond automatically when the self-image, or sense of who we are (whether false or real), is being attacked. Early programming thus evolves into a repetitive, response pattern in later life, reinforcing Berne's life script theory. Through these servo-mechanisms, whenever the ego perceives it needs protection the programming kicks in and goes on automatic, the learned signals are transmitted to the brain, and the closed feedback loop again serves its master.

Admittedly, early programming sustained by ego defense mechanisms is often a survival strategy appropriate for the time it was designed but not for old age. The needs of elders and circumstances change, and one of the tasks of old age is to transcend the ego controls and fixations, not to expand or reinforce them. Until the courage is found to let go of the perceived self-illusions and reach for the true Self, toxic agers are compelled to keep their defense mechanisms in order to protect their false images. Unfortunately, by holding on to that protection, old distorted feelings and *maladaptive* solutions are perpetually retaped in a closed toxic loop.

Kinds of Defense Mechanisms

Of the many defense mechanisms identified, the most visibly employed by toxic agers are as follows (see the Glossary for DSM-IV [APA, 1994] expanded definitions):

Denial of reality—used adroitly to evade owning painful inner feelings and behavior in order to avoid confronting and working through internal resentments, anger, fear, and guilt. This denial can also draw a family into a sense of collusion and co-Victim toxicity.

Projection—placing what is not acceptable in oneself onto others. If the projections are taken on by others, the toxic agers are now free to blame the receivers for the very things the toxics despise in themselves. The recipients have become the toxics denied mirror.

Reaction Formation—a self-serving form of conscious behavior or attitude that is executed in direct opposition to usual patterns of behavior, such as a toxic's smile and charming interchange with outsiders to mislead and manipulate their environment.

Counterattack—an attack usually aimed at those closest to the toxics when, in actuality, they are angry at themselves and unable to accept and own the fear behind their anger. By shifting the blame the fears are displaced.

Repression—often used by toxics to push down and block out the unacceptable bad feelings or impulses that they refuse to see or own or are unable to express.

Withdrawal—usually a passive-aggressive silent treatment or self-righteous martyrdom, with secret gloating over the frustration they cause.

Control Theory

During the late 1930s, scientists in a variety of fields were becoming interested in designing control devices that would enable humans to act on their world instead of reacting to its external forces. Especially interested were some of the research theorists in cybernetics who recognized that feedback was essential in making control systems work. One admirer of these men was William T. Powers, a physicist and engineer, who wrote *Behavior: The Control of Perception* (1973). William Glasser, the founder of Reality Therapy, was so enamored with the concept of behavioral control through perception that he wrote two books on control theory based on Powers's work (1981, 1985).

In the foreword to Glasser's (1981) first book on control theory, Powers summed up the essence of his theory by stating the basic premise: "We control what we perceive, not what actually exists, and not what we do." In other words, we maintain balance by selectively inhibiting outside stimuli from entering our brain if they do not match our internal perceived needs, values, and wants. By doing this, a behavioral response is generated from inside to correlate with the pictures or images we have in our heads.

As I understand this complex process, if we visualize in our minds that our needs and wants are satisfied, whether self-destructive or constructive, we have the perception of being in control. This means, according to Glasser, that with this kind of power, even though it may be an illusion, we have the ability to choose our own misery or joy, what we subject ourselves to, and what we put into our computer-like brains.

Interestingly, this is the same thread, and message, pervasive in the basic theoretical assumptions of this text, in the concept of scripts in TA, and in the cognitive psychology of Responsible Assertion training (see chapter 10). If we change our thinking, shift our perceptions, and choose to act accordingly, we have the power to rewrite our own life script, stop or continue the psychological games, and be in control of how we respond to outside situations or stimuli. That is personal power, incomprehensible to toxic agers. They only know, deep inside, that they are not satisfied. Consequently, they play Control, a game that gives them the illusion of power.

Cybernetics and Psychocybernetics

Surprisingly, additional support for the theories previously described was accidentally discovered when conducting the literature search for causes of toxicity, and seemed fundamental in validating the integration concept of Nature and Nurture.

As early as the 1940s and 1950s, 30 of the best minds in the world met yearly in Chicago and in Belgium to construct a new and practical gestalt framework that would provide a universal explanation of life itself—in a sense a new paradigm. Participants were from multiple disciplines such as physics, math, computer science, neurophysiology, and psychiatry and included such persons as Gregory Bateson, Margaret Mead, Norbert Wiener, Warren McCulloch, and Heinz von Foerster. Their goal was to find a fresh interdisciplinary language that would enable them to construct a unifying system that explained how life was organized, how the brain worked, and how to analyze complicated behavioral and information-processing systems. After years of critiquing and testing their ideas, they called their system "Cybernetics," Greek for steersmanship (Maltz, 1969).

The idea of "steering" came from the determination that the subconscious was actually the brain, and the nervous system was controlled and operated by the mind to steer us toward a specified goal. Maltz called this steering a "servo-mechanism, an automatic goal-seeking machine which steers itself to a target or goal through use of feedback data and stored information, automatically correcting the course when necessary" (1969, pp. 40–41). He also wanted to make it very clear that human beings were not machines but that the brain and body function as a computer-type system that responds when turned on with given input. Eventually, this input becomes automatic (and subconscious) when an error-free approach is finally discovered after many corrective, interactive feedback trials. Since the brain cannot discern whether the input is factual or imaginary, a mental image pictured in the mind is enough to trigger the automatic response and the desired results.

Although Maltz wrote mostly about the positive outcomes of his servo-mechanisms, it follows that the input given this automatic system could be negative. If so, and if the closed feedback loop, a key component of cybernetic thinking, is eventually locked into this negativity, the outcomes would also be negative—the explanation for the toxic loop.

It appears that, over time, toxic agers have locked themselves into an automatic, and closed, negative feedback system that perpetually feeds on itself, steering unaware agers through an endless toxic loop. This also means, as stated earlier by Gurdjieff, that it would take a heavy shock to the system to intervene and stop the habituated cycle.

The Internal Environment

For toxic agers, the feedback loops become negative response patterns that match the type of early data and emotions they have put into the internal system. For example, their negative self-talk tapes play loudly and constantly in their heads, causing a projected, negative reaction to their environment.

This thinking is also reinforced by neurobiological studies and the response patterns of the body cell receptors to the chemical peptides that transmit the emotions. In a sense, the interaction has "transformed mind into matter" (Pert quoted in Chopra, 1997, p. 3), with emotions as the connecting link between both, whether negative or positive.

Summary

Chapter 10 contains a variety of theories that support the dual Nature and Nurture concept as being instrumental in developing the personality and the character. It is the response patterns in interaction between individuals and their environment—the internal and external forces—that shape the attitudes and behaviors displayed. Both are significant. Finding an integrated balance is attainable for successful agers but seemingly unreachable for toxic agers. For them, the inner tension between what they perceive nature and nurture should be but are not is constant and fearful.

Several specific theories of TA are presented to demonstrate the interactive dynamics between individual choice and environmental impact. They are as follows:

- Life Script—its correlation to Victimization
- Stroking—to prevent emotional deprivation
- Ego States—for identifying personality subparts
- Games and Karpman's Triangle—to analyze and understand unconscious transactions between ego states that further the script

Reference to Bowlby's Attachment Theory is also made to emphasize his thesis that if the need to love and be loved is blocked in childhood, and no intimate bonding occurs, creation of cruel behavior in adults can be the result.

Defense mechanisms are included to show why they are constantly and skillfully used by toxic agers as a means to protect their distorted ego images and maintain the toxicity.

Control Theory states that we control what we perceive, not what actually is, explaining how toxic agers can block outside stimuli and select only that which matches their internal self-illusions, "shoulds," fears, and disintegration.

Cybernetics paints a vivid picture of a closed, feedback loop system and its perpetual cycling. Here, the individual involved (the toxic ager) is stuck in a rigid loop that is closed to input from the outside environment, making the integration of Nature and Nurture unlikely. This concept is reinforced by neurobiological studies that demonstrate that wholeness seems to occur best when Nature and Nurture are connected, when the systems, together with the emotional chemicals, become one.

Part IV

Can We Intervene and Cope? Uncover Negative Beliefs?

The GIFT of happiness belongs to those who unwrap it!

—Author unknown

Chapter 11

Professional Tips

I can't handle it any longer,
came the words of the adult child crying in
your office.

I'm at my wit's end!

Please, help me!

*If only someone would understand! If only there
were some answers, some suggestions, some
solutions . . .*

Depressed, angry, guilty, discouraged, full of disturbing feelings, resentful, and totally drained of all energy, this daughter of a toxic ager is desperate. She is not your client. You did not invite her in. What are you going to do? What is your responsibility? Can you serve her?

Yes, you can serve her. You make the time. At that moment, you are it. You are responsible. It is called crisis intervention. Anyone so full of frustration and anger is a high risk for elder abuse. Verbal, emotional, physical, and even fiduciary abuse are unsurprising by-products when a care provider's situation and exhaustion have pushed him or her beyond personal stress limits and control.

Healthy people avoid toxics if they can. Healthy people refuse to take on the emotional pain. They refuse to submit themselves to the daily complaints, attacks, and ego defenses. They refuse to allow themselves to be contaminated by another's toxicity. Healthy people have learned, usually the hard way, how toxic behavior, thoughts, emotions, and attitudes can create internal tensions, illness, and physical and mental breakdown, a concept so well reinforced by Christiane Northrup (July 1996). Northrup further amplifies this concept by stating, "According to new research, toxic emotions are a key factor in the development of cancers, heart disease, arthritis, and strokes" (p. 3).

Therefore, when adult children walk out on a toxic parent, although it appears to be cold and irresponsible, it may be understandable. It is likely survival. They have had it. For you, however, a professional and service provider, perhaps also a care provider, walking out is not an option. Working with older adults is your job. Some of your clients will be toxic. Many have no family. If they do, you will likely meet the family co-Victim. Although not designated as part of your caseload, if you really want to be effective with your toxic client and provide more than crisis intervention, include the family co-Victim care provider in your treatment plans.

It is possible that, as a professional in the gerontology field, the concept of toxic agers is new to you. If so, your first task is to understand what you are dealing with, be alert to the symptoms of toxicity, seek knowledgeable professional support (ideally a group), learn and use appropriate techniques, maintain the balance between caring involvement and professional detachment, be firm, and remember to apply tough love. Above all, if you happen to also be the child of a toxic ager, be aware of your own toxic predisposition. Accept and work through any hidden tendencies that might interfere with objective help and foster countertransference. If this is not feasible, refer your toxic client to someone else.

These are all critical points, yet the most important one for working with toxic clients, whether they are an aged parent or a 60-year-old adult child (who may also be toxic), is to take care of yourself. This means daily self-nourishment and wellness practices in order to maintain high self-esteem and confidence. That is the most effective way to avoid hooking into the toxic games. As one ombudsman stated, "After years of trial and error, I finally began to realize that the best way for me to help my client was to be self-assured, and to set my own boundaries."

Treatment

I use the term treatment loosely, as toxicity is not treatable in the traditional sense of the medical model cure. Toxic agers cannot be fixed. Once the toxicity is advanced, the pattern is so habituated and suppressed by the toxic ager, that denial prevents a cure. If any healing is to take place, it must come from within the toxic agers themselves, together with an unlikely strong desire and motivation to make the effort (see chapter 13).

If there is treatment, it is best facilitated through the adult children care providers. They have the power and the opportunity to interrupt the co-Victim toxic game feedback loop. By disciplining themselves daily to stop the games (it takes two to play) and to respond differently to their parents' hooks, these adult children can jolt the interactive behavior pattern. This takes effort, determination, and persistence, but with professional support and guidance, adult children care providers are in the unique position to begin to break the destructive transactions, reduce their negative impact, and thus possibly intervene in the passage of toxicity on to the third generation.

Training

Because traditional professional training has not addressed toxicity specifically in older adults, tips were sought from seasoned professionals in the field who were willing to share what they had learned from years of experience with toxic agers. The tips came in the form of insights, usable ideas, and information, as well as specific techniques that generally worked in coping with and setting limits and boundaries for working with toxic agers.

My caution is to remember that each toxic ager is unique. Therefore, the job of service providers, and anyone challenged by these emotionally abusive agers, is to experiment until techniques are found that work for the agers, yourself, your personality, and the personality and degree of disintegration of the toxic ager being dealt with.

Basic Rules

Fundamental to working with toxic agers are three rules:

- Know thyself
- Know what you are dealing with
- Know some intervention tips

Know Thyself

Before you work with toxic agers, check out your own background. I did not. It never occurred to me that 35 years of professional training and experience in how to protect myself were not sufficient when dealing with toxic agers. It seemed impossible that my own vulnerability as the daughter of a toxic would make me so susceptible, albeit unconsciously, to the toxicity.

As I reflect on my career, I am aware of how different it might have been if I had known about toxicity, what I was dealing with, and my own toxic tendencies. Instead of being a co-Victim and perpetuating my mother's toxicity, I could have shifted my perceptions, seen and responded to her as a client instead of my mother, and emotionally disengaged. Perhaps then, objectivity would have returned. Being unaware, however, hooking into the games was inevitable. I had perfected too many years of practice in being part of the toxic loop. As a daughter, I was just as susceptible to the toxic games as anyone else. Professional training was no cure. I did not know myself or what it meant to be toxic.

I was not alone, however. For example, one of the MFCCs I interviewed for this book (chapter 5) told me of two social worker friends of hers who were daughters of toxic mothers. Relief for the first friend came only after her mother died and the game triangle was broken. The situation had become so bad that the social worker was unable to work for an entire month.

The second friend, a recent graduate with a degree in social work, had desperately tried to please her mother and make her happy, using all her knowledge and training. Nothing seemed to work. The guilt she felt worsened her feelings of helplessness, especially when she could not talk about it. As a professional, she assumed she should know how to handle the situation; instead, she was only too aware of her own depleted energy.

Know What You Are Dealing with

Understand Your Client

Toxic agers seek attention when they discover that their old ways of negative coping and controlled manipulation, the only strategies they know, are no longer effective. Then comes the realization that they are also unable to manage their feelings. Because they are too rigid to change, toxic agers act like fearful children and either lash out or withdraw into their own despair. The question is, when do you intervene and, if so, how?

Levels of Dysfunction

Before any action is undertaken, careful discernment of the type of dysfunction should be made. Difficult behaviors can be divided into three levels:

1. *Adjustment Problems:* symptoms of grief, depression, anxiety, physical complaints, anger, withdrawal, or conduct problems; usually the result of the inability to adapt within a reasonable period of time after a traumatic event, significant loss, or some identifiable psychosocial stressor.

   This is *not* toxicity and can be treated with traditional approaches, such as empathy, active listening, case management, peer counseling, workshops, or a support group.

2. *Lifelong Maladaptation or Toxicity:* patterns of Victim consciousness formed from early negative interactions between significant, childhood environmental forces and an innate personality tendency toward toxicity. Most traditional approaches are ineffective.

3. *Personality Disorders:* primarily DSM-IV (APA, 1994) diagnostic classifications, such as paranoid, borderline, schizoid, antisocial, histrionic, and obsessive-compulsive, that require psychotherapy and medication.

Clarity concerning what you are working with is the essential first step, followed by knowing what you can do, how you will maintain it, and then doing it with confidence.

Basic Guidelines

The best way to understand what we as professionals, caregivers, and adult children care providers in the gerontology field are facing in our work with toxic agers is to remind ourselves, again, of some basic givens.

1. *Manage or cope; don't try to "fix" a toxic ager.* Toxic turmoil is within. It is not a physiological ailment but a negative psychic energy. It is a destructive force of Victim consciousness that can ultimately consume both the toxic ager and the person(s) psychologically entrapped in its influence. Dissipation is possible if the toxicity is brought into conscious awareness. Without the toxic agers themselves acknowledging, owning, embracing, and integrating their toxicity, however, the possibility that they will become whole and achieve inner peace is doubtful.

2. *Realize all possess both toxic and nourishing qualities.* According to Greenwald's theory (1969), all individuals have internal, unique, intrapsychic patterns that enable them to self-generate either nourishing or toxic behavior. In other words, we all have a choice in how we respond to life: either with self-nourishment or self-toxification.

3. *Shift your perception of toxic agers—it is key.* Granted, it will take continuous effort, but until you can shift your perception of toxic clients and see them as a challenge from which you can learn, like an adventure for growth, they will remain a problem that will not go away.

4. *Understand what it means to deal with toxics.* Because you are dealing with "shadow energy," accept the fact that visible results will be minimal. You are *not* responsible for the toxic's choice of behavior or emotions. By using professional detachment you can maintain an objective balance, showing you care but without personal entanglement.

5. *Avoid the "hook" of the psychological toxic games.* Psychological games take two people to play. Whether unconscious or not, if you get hooked and play, you are just as responsible as the toxic ager.

6. *Don't be a sucker for a "guilt trip."* Toxics are well-known for placing guilt trips on anyone open to their entrapment. It is called, "Poor Me—Gotcha"; an emotionally seductive game. Be alert for these passive-aggressive manipulations. Psychological guilt is a choice.

7. *Never try to "make" a toxic ager feel happy.* Happiness is self-induced. Trying to *make* another happy is hopeless. If taken on, it will magnify into a vicious cycle of effort and rejection, especially with full-blown toxic agers.

8. *Remind yourself that your most important task is consistent, daily self-nourishment.* It does not take much to realize that if you are "down," stressed-out, angry, or pushed to the limit, you will not be able to handle any true toxic (aged or not). Check the chapter on self-help for some specific self-nourishment techniques.

9. *Appreciate that probably the foremost ingredient toxic agers need is "unconditional love."* Toxic agers are desperate for unconditional love, but they do not know it. Ironically, they make it almost impossible for others to love them, rejecting all

positive strokes in order to maintain their negative energy and life script. Love them anyway. Unconditional love needs no return, and it will have an impact.

Know Some Intervention Tips

Often, the wisest approach you can have is to observe, listen to, and learn from other professionals active in the field. Below are some valuable tips that are usable and practical. Additional strategies and techniques will be discussed in chapter 12.

Tips from Feil's Validation Method

Over the years Feil (1992a) developed many effective methods for working with deteriorating and difficult old-old adults, classifying their behavior in various stages (see chapter 9 on theories).

Most of Feil's clients have progressed beyond the preliminary stage that she and Erikson called the stage of maladaptation (and I call early toxicity) to the stage of malorientation. Because the maloriented stage of unfinished development parallels that of the advanced stage of toxicity in older adults, Feil's tips on working with the maloriented old-old become wise professional guides for working with toxic agers.

As I understand them, these guides are as follows:

1. Foremost: respect that the maloriented (or toxics) *must* initiate their own healing process. They cannot be fixed is a phrase I use often.
2. When working with maloriented (or toxics), first acknowledge to yourself your own hurt or disgust, then put it aside and get on with the work.
3. Center yourself. Clear out your own feelings.
4. Take the maloriented (or toxics) where they are; then identify who they are. Say to yourself, "Oh, a Blamer" or "a Whiner." This tactic will enhance the understanding of the person you are dealing with and facilitate the sorting process regarding the type of approach to use.

5. Pay close attention to the nonverbals of the maloriented client (or the toxic ager). Because their skill at using verbal defense mechanisms are so practiced, their body language is the best indicator of what is going on inside. Be alert for the messages available through the pitch, volume, and speed of the voice; facial expressions; body movement; and gestures. This kind of observation is one of the best ways to break through the armor.
6. Don't ask questions. LISTEN! OBSERVE!
7. Search for something real inside the maloriented (or toxic) with which to work.
8. Never lie to them. Mean what you say.
9. Be gentle but strong. Set firm limits, then stick to them. The maloriented (and toxics) respect personal power.
10. Model coping techniques, not just for the maloriented (or toxic agers) but for others who have to deal with them.
11. Do *not* suggest group therapy or support groups. Maloriented (or toxics) are unable to deal with feelings and would only manipulate or destroy the group. One to one works best. If they are in the early stages and still active, however, a political- or issue-oriented group may work because their anger energy can be productively transferred to an outside issue.

Tips from the Recovery Movement

To deal with the confused boundaries of toxic agers and establish limits to their invasive behavior, Love (1990) designed an assertion technique she calls the "Ten-Second Confrontation," which may work with toxic clients. The process consists of making confronting statements that are brief, specific, honest, direct, clear, appropriate, and responsible. As Love says, you "make your point, then get off it" (1990, p. 2). The key is that all of these "points" must be made in a firm, calm, steady voice and with congruent body language so that the receiver knows immediately that what is said is meant.

Because toxic agers are not used to people assertively standing up to them, you may be tested to see if you mean what you say.

If they resist, apply the "broken record" assertion skill. Simply repeat or paraphrase the statement with a firm voice and convincing body language while looking the client straight in the eye. If they persist after three repeats or start getting angry, just shift to a different approach.

The following are some examples of possible confrontational statements that your clients will respect if they sense you care. It is best, however, to develop your own words.

- Martha, it seems as if all you want to do is confuse the issue. I will reschedule our appointment for next Wednesday, when we can make some decisions.
- With a toxic client who is complaining with excessive loudness, interrupt by calling him by name and saying firmly, "Randolph, you have been complaining very loudly for 15 minutes now. It is making it difficult for me to hear what you want from me. Here's a pencil and some paper. Make a list of what you want. I'll be back in 5 minutes, and then we can work it out."
- If the client contact is the third or more phone call of derogatory comments about your abilities, politely, but firmly, say, "I'm sorry you feel that way. I'll refer you to my supervisor. Just a moment please . . . " and then quickly call your supervisor and prep him or her for the situation. Whenever working with a toxic ager, always inform your supervisor in advance and work out a strategy. Team support with toxics is critical.

Also, when working with toxic agers, do not expect immediate results. Change in realigning your relationship will take time, patience, experimentation, and risk. In addition, make sure your supervisor understands what you are dealing with so you do not feel pressured to produce unrealistic outcomes. Work with all the client's interactive systems, such as family and senior centers, in order to block the toxic ager from finding other game players. In the long run, this endeavor will pay off, if you're permitted to do more than crisis intervention.

Tips from Service Providers

Seasoned professionals and service providers from a variety of different areas (see chapter 5) in the gerontology field were glad to share some tips learned over years of trial and error in hopes it would prevent others from experiencing the same anguish they felt in the early days of their careers. Because many of those interviewed were connected to senior centers, public services, and groupings of older adults, the initial common practice with toxic agers was to contain the distractions. It was more expedient to avoid, circumvent, block, or simply remove the offending ager from the premises. In advanced cases, even today, these tactics may be reverted to, when everything else fails, and it is simply too time consuming, draining, and detracting from other participants.

To be truly effective with the most difficult agers, however, it often takes years of learning the toxics' patterns, gaining their trust, and experimenting until something is found that works for each particular person. Because individual agers respond differently, as do professionals, solutions must vary according to the personalities and situations involved and the intensity and frequency of contact. The essential element for all, however, is the practice of immediately establishing consistent and firm ground rules, plus setting and maintaining clear boundaries, strategies that advocate the relevancy of prevention.

The following words from these seasoned service providers are best called sage advice:

- First, get a firm grip on your own anger.
- Be direct, to the point, and take control.
- Don't spend time and energy trying to reason with them [toxic agers].
- Be firm, set limits, talk sternly if you have to.
- Center yourself.
- Acknowledge who they are. "Oh, that's Edna!"
- Let them talk enough so they feel they have had their say or, in other words, let them run down to dissipate the negative energy.
- Do not perceive yourself as being the cause of their problems, avoid taking their outbursts personally.
- Keep yourself detached enough so you do not get personally involved and lose your objectivity.
- Remember they will "crunch" you as well as themselves . . . they have no capacity for any insight.

- Take time out, walk away if necessary, and if possible.
- Arrange with another worker to deal with them if you are having a bad day.
- Find their interests, try to assimilate them, or give them "real" work off by themselves.
- Make frequent changes in the volunteers or staff who have to work with them.
- If they come in mad and frustrated, get them off by themselves, try to find out what the problem is, and see to it they get to the proper resource.
- Help staff to understand what they are dealing with and handle with gentle firmness.
- Make it very clear to them the type of behavior that is acceptable and not acceptable.
- If in a group, keep the group highly structured with firmly set ground rules.
- If they do not adhere to appropriate behavior standards and refuse to treat others with kindness, ask them to come to your office, and in a one-to-one setting, with a soft firm voice, explain that that kind of behavior will not be tolerated. If it continues they will not be allowed to return. If they show up anyway, it is OK to call the police as a last resort.
- Allow peer pressure to work. Other seniors will often not tolerate negative behavior.
- Protect others in the program. Confront toxics privately, in a firm but loving way, so they know you mean business if they do not treat others with respect. Either they shape up, or they do not get the service.
- Institute an Advisory Council made up of 15 to 20 seniors in the program who will counsel on personality problems that arise. The toxics are given a one-to-one warning. If mistreatment to others continues, the toxic goes before the Council. (Note: this may not work with advanced toxicity.)
- Document incidences; know your facts; be very specific and frank with dates, times, places, and witnesses when confronting the toxic ager about inappropriate behavior.
- Keep your Board well-appraised of any problems with toxics. Toxics are the first to write or telephone in complaints, as well as stir up negative evaluations. Feeling intimidated or fearful of this type of person can be deadly.

- Get yourself a professional support group to keep up your own self-esteem when first starting out, especially if your Center happens to be blessed with a plethora of toxics.
- Do not personalize their behavior, do not argue, and always remember to use humor. Unless the toxicity is advanced, light teasing works wonders.

After reading these suggestions, I hope you found them as helpful as I did. It is pure agony and time consuming to work this out on your own. All of the long-term senior center directors admitted it was extremely difficult in the beginning. The toxic agers were very intimidating. It was not until the directors attained a sense of certainty within themselves and were able to keep their own self-confidence and esteem up that they felt their own effectiveness. With toxics, one learns to dig deep inside to find personal resources never before known to exist.

Transactional Analysis Tips

TA is an old model and much covered in the last chapter, but because I still find it to be one of the most helpful and practical approaches to working with toxic agers, I am including a synopsis of the key concepts. For a deeper understanding of the theory, I recommend James and Jongeward's classic, *Born to Win* (1973). It is also a good referral for the adult children. It will provide a theoretical base to help you understand the dynamics between yourself and your client and some possible reasons for the behavior and transactions that occur.

The TA concepts most applicable for practical use are as follows:

Positive Stroking, or Warm Fuzzies. Professionally known as "units of recognition or love," warm fuzzies are ways to affirm, nourish, and rebuild self-esteem—critical for you as professionals, the toxic ager, and adult children co-Victims. Based on spiritual love, warm fuzzies are a path to healing. If genuine, appropriate, timely, and responsible, they are extremely effective. Examples are a warm smile, a hug, a touch, a thoughtful gesture, attentiveness, meaningful notes or looks, a phone call, personal time, or the two most significant fuzzies: active listening and your personal presence; just being there for the other. The key? Remembering to give them to yourself, coworkers, and others—daily.

Life Scripts. Awareness of the types of negative scripts written by small children helps in grasping, with some clarity, the lifetime of human dramas the toxic agers unconsciously play out. It also alerts us to the professional support it would take to break through the ego defenses and games that maintain the Victimization and closed toxic loop, even if the toxic ager chooses (which is doubtful) to rewrite the script.

Ego States. Identification of subpersonality type patterns (Parent, Adult, and Child) is essential in helping us, as professionals, to discern which ego state we need to employ in order to effectively connect with the toxic ager's operating ego state and get our message through. Problem solving, unfortunately, is negligible because the Adult ego state of the toxic is underdeveloped. This leaves you, essentially, working primarily from your Nurturing Parent.

This means making statements to clients with a mixture of firmness and caring. It is called "tough love." The reason? When toxic agers are acting like whining, complaining, or rebellious children you have only two choices for communicating in a way that will reach them in their Child ego state: either the Parent ego state (Critical or Nurturing,) or the comparable Child ego state that is neither effective nor professional. (Review the TA section in chapter 10.)

Psychological Game Playing. Passive-aggressive game playing is about the only way toxics interact, thinking they are communicating. As a professional, your task is to recognize the games and avoid the entrapments. If you suddenly realize you are hooked and in your Child ego state, concede your involvement, and then shift to, and stay in, your Adult ego state. This action will automatically stop the game. Why? Because the objective, unemotional, rational Adult in all of us does not play games.

Another technique for stopping a game is to give unexpected answers (such as agreeing with the toxic ager, called fogging in assertion training), which will leave your client momentarily speechless and enable you to redirect the transaction or, as in the case of one social worker's response, stop the game. When she asked a toxic client why his children did not visit, his brusque response was, "I don't want to see my kids." Her immediate rejoinder was, "Oh, you really want to see them!" Whereupon he stopped, then opened up. (See Game Stopping on pages 230–231.)

Responsible Assertion Training Tips

Probably one of the most effective skills for anyone working with toxic or difficult agers is another model initiated in the 1970s that is also still operative and relevant to toxic agers. It is called Responsible Assertion Training (discussed in detail in chapter 12). Assertion workshops or classes can still be found in community service programs, but before signing up, be sure to check out the value system of the approach. Look for what is called "Responsible Assertion," because some assertion training is amoral. A manipulative, aggressive, attack approach would negate any productive work with toxics. The best resources are *Responsible Assertive Behavior* (Lange & Jakobowski, 1976), which is geared to potential trainers of the system, and *Assertive Options* (Jakobowski & Lange, 1979), an excellent resource for students.

Responsible Assertion Training not only teaches coping skills and techniques for working with difficult people, but also helps to build self-esteem and assurance, which in turn discourages game playing. When used effectively, toxics quickly get the message that assertors mean what they say and won't be manipulated. It also teaches the importance of recognizing the passive-aggressiveness in toxic behavior, the most challenging, guilt-inducing style to deal with.

In addition, being assertive does not mean that assertors get everything they want. Instead it means that they are clear on what they need or want, have the ability to be brief and succinct in asking for it, and express their thoughts and feelings appropriately, firmly, and responsibly.

An example of such clarity and honest appropriate expression was shared by an ombudsman who also happened to be the daughter of a toxic father, as well as having worked with 40 to 50 toxics over the previous 10 years. One day, when one of her toxic clients was being quite loud and gruff (she had just placed him in his fifth Board and Care in 3 weeks), she looked him in the eye and quietly but firmly said, "You act like a mean old man. I've been raised by a mean man, so you don't scare me." Whereupon, he melted.

Typical of other incidences, this professional had learned that if she stood up to these toxic agers, was honest and straight with them, acted with love, and did not "wimp under," they would respect her. In fact, in practicing responsible assertiveness, she found that these clients often said to her, "You're the only one who cares." But, she warned, if a worker doesn't keep herself separate so as not to get caught up in their intimidations, "they literally kill us."

Time Out. Highly useful in certain situations, time out will give both you and your client a chance to reduce the tension levels. When it does not work, just cancel the session and set another time. It is essential for you to maintain control and to establish a productive climate and consistent pattern when working with a toxic ager. In essence you are training him or her how to respond to you, not vice versa.

Assimilating the skills of responsible assertion, however, takes more than reading a book. Mastering the techniques of cognitive restructuring, behavioral rehearsal or role playing, and coaching takes time and persistent practice, which will be discussed in chapter 12, Strategies and Techniques.

Summary

Pearls of wisdom were sought from a variety of professionals, researchers, authors, and seasoned service providers with years of experience to ascertain the best ways to work with toxic agers. Their collective advice was as follows:

- Understand what you are dealing with
- Learn, and use, appropriate techniques
- Maintain balance and detachment

- Be firm and apply tough love
- Watch for any predispositions toward toxicity in yourself, especially if a child of a toxic
- Never forget to nourish yourself daily

Traditional treatment with toxic agers is not feasible. They cannot be fixed. Coping and interrupting the toxic game loop are the best approaches. Any healing must come from within the toxics themselves.

Specialized training in toxicity is helpful. Three basic rules support professional advice:

1. Know thyself.
2. Know what you are dealing with.
3. Know the intervention techniques that work.

Described also are the 3 levels of dysfunction, 9 givens as to what to expect with toxic agers, 11 tips from Feil's Validation method, Love's "One Minute Confrontation" assertion approach, valuable advice from veteran service providers, and practical TA tips on how to use warm fuzzy strokes, life scripts, ego states, and game playing.

Responsible Assertion Training is introduced, with a few examples of its professional value. Behavioral rehearsal or role playing, cognitive restructuring, and coaching techniques will be reviewed in the next chapter.

In essence, the ideal is for gerontology professionals to recognize what they are dealing with and to be a catalyst for preventing toxicity from infiltrating and destroying the positiveness of an aging process that nature meant to be beautiful and successful.

Chapter 12

Strategies and Techniques

Caution is the word when using techniques. They are presented here only as possible supplemental tools, not as treatment. The key component in working with toxic clients is yourself, your own beingness. The ideal is to be fully attuned and present, a model of healing love. The ability to see value in these agers, gain their trust, show you care nonverbally, look for the spiritual love deep inside them, and still be tough is what will make the difference. Strategies and techniques are only tactics to open the process, a place to start. Use them wisely.

Remember, with toxicity you are dealing with externalized symptoms of inner unconscious conflicts and fear. They are so suppressed it will take a shock to awaken the toxic agers enough for them to want to change, an action usually too fearful for them to attempt. Consequently, work with toxics is usually that of containment, setting limits, avoiding the toxic games, and dealing with the co-Victim adult child. For real healing to even begin, it takes a shift in perception, a shift from seeing the toxic agers as frustrating problems to seeing them as a new adventure. In this adventure you, and those affected by toxic agers, can grow. In this adventure difficulties become an opportunity, not a burden. In this adventure the toxics themselves become your best teacher.

Structured Intervention

Because I feel so certain about the healing power of perceptual shifts, I caution against the use of the family intervention technique (similar to that used with alcoholics) for toxic agers. It may well be the shock some ingrained toxics need. It is definitely an effective, confrontational method if done in love and will clarify a relationship. I wonder, however, how successful this type of intervention is with older, more advanced toxic agers (and their co-Victims trapped in Victim consciousness and toxic game loops) particularly when we are reminded that it takes at least two to play the toxic game.

Nevertheless, a structured intervention can be a potent last-resort tool. If there is extensive preparation; it is highly organized; all significant relationships are committed, participating, fully in agreement, and trained; it is appropriate and feasible for that particular toxic ager—then the strategy is professionally facilitated.

Structured intervention is a process that forces adult children to face up to their collective fears, confront their parents with the truth, and possibly break the toxic pattern and cycle so it is not passed on to the grandchildren. This is laudable. There are two questions, however. When it involves toxic agers, can we assume the co-Victim can refrain from reentering the toxic games, and is the risk worth the effort? The manipulative skills of advanced toxics are so honed, they are likely to infect the process; turn it around; become the martyr; and leave the adult children, especially the co-Victim, with unbearable guilt. Education then appears to be the most appropriate intervention.

Workshops

Because most toxic agers still resist, reject, and block any visible therapeutic help, direct treatment is usually not effective, nor is it recommended unless desired and requested by the toxic agers themselves. Consequently, the challenge becomes educating those enmeshed in toxic relationships, especially the adult children and co-Victims who help perpetuate the interlocking toxic games and system. Others to be reached are professionals (particularly those who are adult children of toxic parents), older adults who fear they might become toxic, and early-stage toxic agers. With such a variety of potential students, the most effective way "to give away what we know, to teach people to help themselves and others," is probably through workshops (Schlossberg, 1990, p. 9).

Content of these workshops is best developed in accord with the particular needs of each group. A variety of interactive strategies, techniques, and group processes such as self-protective social skills, TA, assertion training, self-esteem building, stress management, self-nourishment, and wellness practices work best.

If the workshop is made up of early-stage toxic agers, however, make certain they have identified and owned their toxicity, want the experience, and are ready to face themselves. Do not undertake this group unless these agers acknowledge that they are the cause of their behavior, accept their role and responsibility, commit themselves to changing their habits, show that they are willing to make the effort to learn to love, and are able to trust and feel safe with a strong and caring facilitator or counselor.

Gerontology professionals and older adults eager to prevent toxicity are easy to work with. The group presenting the greatest challenge and need, however, is the adult children, especially if they are co-Victims. They provide the opportunity for you to have an impact on relieving guilt and frustration, as well as breaking the generational toxic cycle. With the interruption of the negative pattern, you can facilitate a coordinated effort with the adult children that will benefit them, their parents, and your clients.

Workshop Structure

The framework and time of the workshops are best designed to meet the needs and convenience of both you and the students, ranging from 2-hour seminars to 12-week classes. My personal preference is a combination workshop and support group, scheduled as two 6-week series. Meeting once a week, each session would consist of 3 hours, with a half-hour break in the middle to enable the natural formation of support networks. I also advise closing the workshop to new members after the first session. Group size seems to work best if maintained between 6 and 10 participants.

Personal interviews prior to a workshop are advantageous, but probably the most important aspect is a 3-month commitment from each participant to attend and work. Reason? I have found that it takes at least 3 months to break old habits and cement changes. Being toxic prone, adult children also have to work on their own toxicity. Therefore, having to report back on their progress each week, especially to a group, is not only helpful but also subtly forces the effort.

Also, if a workshop or support network system related to toxic agers is not available, start one. Few institutions and programs offer more than a brief training on difficult elderly, and nothing on toxic agers. The reduction of strain and frustration would be worth the effort.

Workshop Pattern

One pattern for such a workshop and support group might be Adult Children of Toxic Agers (ACTA), a program I initiated in 1992 in response to a letter received from an adult child of a toxic parent urging that a support group be started to help her and others in her situation.

The acronym ACTA was deliberately used for the group's name because several of the adult children feared that their toxic parents might find out what they were doing. To them, being honest and prompting another tirade was pure stupidity. Besides, another problem was definitely not needed. Partway through the first workshop, however, one daughter was able to say to her mother in a firm, half teasing, but loving way, "I'm going to a class to learn how to get along with you."

With the exception of the first session, the workshop pattern, although flexible, is usually an even division between a support group and a class. The first session is devoted to getting acquainted, laying the ground rules, establishing workshop expectations, building group trust and cohesiveness, and sharing of personal stories. Subsequent sessions open with a stress reduction technique, followed by a 3-minute report from each participant on his or her progress during the week. This progress can be as simple as seeing something positive in a parent or catching themselves and stopping the game before getting hooked. The second half of each session consists of exercises and group processes, the content, a weekly assignment, and feedback of what each learned.

Workshop Content

Ideally, workshop content focuses on understanding toxicity and its challenge, the interactive role of the adult children, personality type theory, the practical application of coping strategies, skills practice, and a chance to test some of the theories. The support group and personal networks will emerge.

Follow-up

An advanced group follow-up session is recommended in 6 to 9 months depending on the expressed needs of the participants. Ongoing, time-limited, support groups are also encouraged, enabling participants who have completed at least the initial 6-week workshop to get support in reinforcing and maintaining learned skills and their confidence and self-love.

Critical to a program of this type is the facilitation of an environment that will enable the participants to share their stories, rebuild their self-esteem, affirm and nourish their inner child, practice self-assertiveness, establish ongoing support linkages, and learn some specific techniques.

Feedback

According to follow-up reports, the ACTA workshops are workable means for reducing frustrations, feelings of guilt, and a deep sense of inadequacy. To adult children of toxic agers, the most comforting part is often knowing that others understand. At last, they are not alone. Sometimes just having a label for the syndrome is helpful. It is common to hear these children say that knowing they are dealing with an emotional poison means they can disassociate and protect themselves without the devouring guilt. Now they can energize enough strength to meet the challenge up front. Adult children who are professionals involved in the program also report extensive improvement in their personal life that usually spills over into their work, making them exceptionally effective with toxic agers.

Results are promising. Workshops and support groups such as ACTA effectively sustain adult children, especially during the initial stages when they assume care providing responsibility for a toxic parent. These groups also help to replace, or support, the extensive individual therapy and medication for depression and suicidal thoughts so prevalent among many of the ACTA participants. Because toxicity is such a hidden phenomenon, however, it is often difficult to find these desperate adult children unless the toxic parent has been brought to the attention of social services. Public awareness and openness are needed. New programs are needed. If there are none where you are, start one.

Forewarnings

When working with toxic co-Victims, as with toxic agers, do not expect any spontaneous remissions. Change and realignment of a relationship take time, patience, experimentation, and risk. As an adult child said to me, "It's slow, but I can see some progress. I'm becoming clearer on what I need and want, am able to express it with appropriate confidence, and to establish limits. I think mother is as surprised as I am."

Also, with many co-Victims you will often find a general grieving over the letting go of old conditioning, behavioral patterns, expectations, and, most of all, the loss of game playing to fill time. Recognize it. It takes many forms, but if a sense of shock, withdrawal, anger, boredom, or depression occurs, help workshop participants understand and own it, feel the pain, and work through it. One of the most difficult perceptions for adult children to let go of is trying to make their toxic parents into the persons they wish they had been, parents who are able to love them. Grief work is mandated when this is finally opened up and accepted.

Resources

Among the referral sources useful for adult children and co-Victims are books from two bestselling authors. In 1973, Jerry Greenwald wrote *Be the Person You Were Meant to Be*. To my knowledge, it was the first book written about toxicity and nourishment. Susan Forward wrote *Toxic Parents: Overcoming Their Hurtful Legacy and Reclaiming Your Life* (1989) and, her latest book, *Emotional Blackmail: When the People in Your Life Use Fear, Obligation and Guilt to Manipulate You* (1997). Although only a few pages are dedicated to elderly parents, the concepts are applicable to all ages and are therefore good adjuncts to this book.

In Part Two of Forward's (1989) book, entitled *Reclaiming Your Life*, she offers specific techniques and strategies for changing self-defeating patterns and shifting from victimization to freedom. This includes specific exercises on how to confront toxic parents, the most difficult, but self-empowering task faced by adult children.

Still, my own bias in facilitating a learning process for adult children of toxic agers is, as expressed by Forward in her epilogue (1989), to "let go of the struggle." For me this means to help adult children and co-Victims take control of their lives, set limits, be firm and assertive, be clear on the relationship, trust themselves, and avoid all psychological game playing. It means encouraging adult children to see their parents as clients or patients, shifting their role from that of emotionally imprisoned children to disengaged professionals who serve with loving care. It means teaching these children to stay in their Adult and Nurturing Parent ego states long enough to respond with objective understanding, not blind subjectivity. It means inspiring them to look for the love and beauty in their parents, making it a new adventure—an exciting challenge.

A Difficult Task

Encouraging adult children to transform their pain into an exciting challenge, however, may turn into your challenge. In researching how adult children typically cope with their parents' toxic behavior, the results show primarily negative coping, essentially attempts to survive. The majority of adult children simply do not have the skills to respond to their environment without getting caught in the toxic web. Consequently, coping strategies vary. Avoidance and escape are the main defenses.

The following are examples of some of the coping tactics used, as stated in the adult children's own words:

I saw as little of her as possible.

I took the phone off the hook.

I bought an answering machine so I wouldn't get stuck listening to her whine and complain.

I kept the discussions superficial and avoided situations that I knew would trigger her wrath. She had a heart condition.

I've learned to lie. I never tell her my true feelings. I also tell her I'm working when I'm not so I'll have at least one day of peace.

None of these adult children felt good about their actions. Guilt was always there. They struggled inside, torn between what they intuitively knew they had to do to survive and what they consciously thought they ought to do as loving, devoted children. They couldn't let go of the struggle, nor could they confront. The tension was agonizing.

One adult child spoke of how, after 50 years, she eventually "solved her problem" by just walking out. There would be no more contacts, no more phone calls—total separation. Thousands of miles established the physical break. The mental and emotional breaks were more difficult, but the distance helped to restore her own sanity. Now, rebuilding her emotional and mental health in a Twelve Step program, she helps frail elderly through a social service agency but still fears her mother's vindictiveness will some-day hurt her.

Negative coping solves nothing. Although it may ease the situation temporarily, the problems always return, seeming worse. Avoidance and distancing may work for strangers, but for family and those ladened with daily contact, the infection only spreads. If allowed to fester, everyone susceptible becomes a co-Victim.

Techniques

It is helpful when facilitating a workshop or support group to have a few suggested techniques at your fingertips. Use what is appropriate for you and your students. It is always best, however, to create your own group processes designed specifically to meet your lesson objectives and purpose.

Perceptual Shift

The concept of perceptual shift has been pervasive throughout this book, but because I feel it is the most powerful, most useful, and first step to healing, I am repeating it here in hopes it will be the foremost approach taught in a workshop or support group geared to breaking the hold of toxicity. My bias is that this hold can be shattered by changing the way we see a person or object, a shift that automatically produces a different response pattern.

That "we respond to things according to the way we perceive them" is an easy concept to understand. The technique, however, is almost too simple; students have a tendency to forget to use it, especially when it is needed the most. Until the shift is internalized, manifested without thought, and emotionally integrated, it takes constant remembering and practice. Exercises help.

Exercise

The purpose here is to shift your students' perception of toxic agers or parents from troublesome, distressing burdens deliberately out to make the students' life miserable to seeing the love and beauty in their toxics. The following steps are suggested.

1. Have your students list all the negative traits of their toxic ager on one half of a sheet of paper.
2. On the opposite half ask them to list all the positive traits.
3. After the students quietly review their own lists, have them write at the bottom what they perceive.
4. Invite each to share, then discuss and process.
5. Now ask the students to close their eyes, visualize that person, and then imagine the fear and hurt behind the individual described on their papers.
6. Next have them visualize their individual as a frightened little girl or boy, unable to trust or feel loved.
7. Talk about the love these children did not get.
8. Now switch to seeing that same child grown up and draw a picture of what they see.
9. Share and process.
10. For the last and key step, invite the students to

    Look for the love and beauty in their agers,

    this time writing what they see and how they feel.
11. Again, follow-up with group processing.

At first there might be some resistance, even tears. That is natural. Attributes that are buried deep are difficult to find. If one persists and looks hard enough and long enough, however, love will seep out. I know. For 2 months, at every visit, I deliberately looked for the love and beauty in my own mother, consciously tuning out her incessant discounts and complaints. During the second month, whenever she started her grievances, I was able to hug her while whispering in her ear, "I love you." By the end of the second month, she finally hugged me back, then whispered "I love you too." This time it was genuine. It seemed like a miracle. Yes, she was my best teacher. At last, I too was beginning to learn to love.

Case Example

Another example of perceptual shift and the value of building self-esteem and confidence was a case presented by a male student of mine, "J," in his early 30's. He was one of three boys, the middle son, who assumed responsibility for his mother when she finally divorced an abusive, controlling husband and had no place to live. It took only a few months after she moved in for the oldest and youngest of the brothers to move out. They could no longer handle her anger, yelling, faultfinding, guilt trips, argumentativeness, and passive-aggressive nagging.

Desperate, and carrying the full load, J went back to school and took my "Assertive Self-Development" class. Over the semester, he was able to build his own self-confidence, esteem himself, learn some skills, and take back his personal power. He shifted his perception of his mother, looked for the love in her, affirmed her daily, set his own boundaries, and practiced assertive skills. She responded, and her behavior changed. She too shifted her perception and began to feel and find love, and finally acceptance, in the local senior center. It must be noted, however, that the toxicity in J's mother was overshadowed by her fear of her husband's overbearing harassment and threats. Under his many years of abuse, her toxicity became noxious, turned inward, and resulted in clinical depression and physical illness. The more typical toxicity did not surface until she was free of her spouse's dominance and ill-treatment and a culture in which women were taught to be submissive. It took time, patience, and J's unconditional love to turn it around, but it worked.

The Goodbye Letter Exercise

Another process that may face resistance and repressed feelings is what I call the "goodbye letter." It is a powerful, viable tool for starting the grief process of "letting go." The letter is to be addressed directly to the toxic parent or ager by name, with the focus on the kind of relationship the professional or adult child perceives they had versus the kind he or she *wishes* they had had, and then say goodbye to them both.

This 15-minute exercise is best facilitated in a support-group atmosphere, *after* group trust and cohesiveness are established. Do not forewarn the attendees. It is easier to tap into their inner Child and spontaneous reactions and repressed feelings if their Critical Parent and ego have not had time to think and control.

Ask the participants to spend the first 12 minutes writing their letters, encouraging them to keep their pens moving constantly, letting their stream of consciousness flow. Suggest they write down all the things they wanted, or wished for, from their toxic parent or significant other but never received, such as support, kind words, attention, encouragement, validation, being there when needed, even material things. This also includes any negative feelings, such as resentment, hurt, anger, or guilt that may be hanging on because of what the toxic ager did to them and, more importantly, what the ager did *not* do.

In the last 3 minutes, students are to write their final goodbye to the perception and image of the parent or person they wished they had. Time is then called. It is helpful to give the students a few minutes to read and reflect on what they have written. In addition, if it seems feasible, a 5-minute break might be appropriate.

Following the break, invite the students to read their letters out loud to the group and, if willing, share what they learned or discovered from the experience. Group members are requested to just listen: no comments, sympathy, or touch, just to affirm and nonverbally project healing love energy, support, and understanding. Hugs are encouraged afterward.

An explanation of the grief process and its stages and the healing components of canceling expectations, forgiveness, and commitment to change may be timely here, depending on the group climate and needs. When completion is felt, group members are usually able to detach enough to see their toxic agers differently, without emotional entanglement, and still be objective and caring. They are ready to accept the same body but will no longer hook into the old toxic games. This is a new person, a new relationship, and a reframed challenge. It is time for the participants to accept their toxic agers as they are—no false perceptions or wishes.

Professionals As Adult Children

For service providers who are also adult children of toxic agers, a goodbye letter can offer an opportunity to bring suppressed emotions and perceptions into awareness. It may be the catalyst that releases the negative energy unconsciously blocking objectivity and effectiveness when dealing with toxic agers, as well as prevent countertransference. As any adult child will tell you, once raised or caught in the toxic loop cycle and game playing, it is a formidable task to break the pattern, almost impossible on your own.

Facilitator Role

One caution regarding using this or other exercises in a workshop. They can be challenging. Before undertaking any group process, you as facilitator must be skilled in group interaction and dynamics, plus sensitive to individual needs, nonverbal signals, level of trust, and readiness of the group.

Transactional Analysis

Much has already been said about TA, but because it is critical in understanding psychological game playing, a key component of toxicity, I need to mention it again. As has been said over and over, it takes two to play a game. Therefore, stopping a game, as one of the professionals I interviewed exclaimed, can be as simple as a one-on-one basketball game. If one of the players steps off the court, the game stops. It is a choice.

Because the perpetuation of toxicity is so dependent on game playing, it is vital that workshop participants be taught early in workshop sessions to recognize their own toxic games, their involvement, and when and how they get hooked. Once recognized, the next step is to know how to stop the games, when and if the players so choose. This skill takes months of practice until identification and game-stopping techniques are automatic. Game hooks are unconscious and will recur endlessly unless avoidance techniques are also habitually ingrained. More details on how to stop a game are presented in the next chapter.

Game Identification Example

The following case scenario is a guide to begin the practice of recognizing games. The games in this case are identified in parentheses as they occur in the example.

The situation referred to came to me via a desperate phone call from a 61-year-old daughter (K), about her 83-year-old toxic mother (L). The tone of the daughter's voice was frustrated, whiny, depressed, and tired. She complained,

> My mother has a heart condition, doesn't drive, and I have to take her to the doctor and shopping. I go see her every day, and it's a 30-mile drive (Poor Me). I'm a Christian, and I'd feel guilty if I didn't (I'm Only Trying To Help) and then when I get there, within 2 minutes we are screaming at each other (Uproar).
>
> I'm like my father, so Mother doesn't like me. I'm an only child. My father died when I was born (Wooden Leg), and I'm the only one mother has. Mother sees and calls herself a victim. She has no friends. I once said I'd kill myself if she died. I didn't mean it, but . . . (Martyr).
>
> I'm a manic-depressive, and on lithium (If It Weren't For . . .).

After a pause, I asked K if she was taking care of herself. Following a moment of silence, she said,

> I know, but I get so worried! (Yes, But . . .)

I then suggested to K that perhaps it would help if she were direct and honest with her mother and told her she'd visit every other day. Without hesitation K's response was,

> Oh no! I can't do that. I'll just say I'm not able to be there (Helpless).

This case may seem extreme. Unfortunately, it is not. It is, instead, a good example of co-Victimization. Until someone wakes up and chooses to stop playing the games, the toxicity in both will unconsciously persist *ad infinitum*. (Explanations of these games can be found in Berne's *Games People Play* (1964) and other TA books.)

Responsible Assertion Training

We have already learned that asking and suggesting do not work with toxic agers. Experience, however, has proved that being skilled in assertion techniques does help in being more effective and self-assured when working with toxic agers in the role of a firm and direct Nurturing Parent. Therefore, it would be wise to teach Responsible Assertion Training (RAT) in all ACTA-type workshops. Also helpful is the clarification of basic personal rights and the practice of specific skills found in all assertion books, such as I messages, stroke and stand, time out, escalation, fogging, and broken record, expressed in detail in chapter 13, p. 228.

For those in frequent contact with toxic agers, time out is a valuable tool. Advise students that it is critical that they insist on time out when tension levels are high and temporarily remove themselves from escalating situations. There is always the promise to return in 5 to 10 minutes when the anxiety is down, and confidence is regained. It is essential that they maintain control and establish a climate and consistent pattern of internal power when working with toxic agers. Remind them often: they are training the toxic ager to respond to them, not vice versa.

My focus here, however, is on three other salient assertion techniques. They are cognitive restructuring, behavior rehearsal, and coaching.

Cognitive Restructuring

Considered part of RAT, cognitive restructuring was derived from the works of Aaron Beck, Stanley Schachter, and Albert Ellis (Lange & Jakobowski, 1976). These cognitive psychologists separately proclaimed that the mind has the power to change and control thinking, feelings, and behavior. According to them, thoughts are the lens through which we see and interpret our world. Judging and labeling determine how we feel and act. As with Control Theory, the general assumption is that a person displays maladjustive behavior because of some error signal or confusion with regard to beliefs and values. There is a "tilt" in the system between what is wanted and expected and what actually is. Neurosis results.

The following vignette is a good example of the need for adult children of toxic agers to become aware of their own automatic self-talk and faulty thinking and to restructure new ways of speaking, thinking, and behaving that are honest and authentic (McKay, Davis, & Fanning, 1981) with their parents.

Vignette

Consider the loving daughter (N), who worries constantly about her elderly toxic mother living alone on the opposite coast. Despite the fact that mother and daughter never got along, N is obsessed with feelings of guilt and agitating self-talk. Relatives and friends reinforce tapes spinning relentlessly in N's head: "You're not a good daughter if you don't take care of your mother. You should bring her out to live with you."

N finally succumbs to her guilt and *insists* that mother come out and live with her. The problem is, mother enjoys her independence and sense of control and doesn't want to move. In her mind, living alone is a symbol of personal power and feelings of worth. N is not aware of her mother's feelings, nor does she realize that as long as mother lives by herself, others can ignore her bitching, complaining, and negativity. Mother, however, likes the martyr role and says nothing to N about how she really feels. She only thinks, "I don't want to hurt my daughter's feelings." A typical avoidance lie that permeates every toxic relation.

So, mother sells her belongings, travels across country, and moves in with N. It does not take long before mother and daughter become co-Victims. Both deteriorate. The close proximity and the mother's loss of control intensify her toxicity and martyrdom. N can no longer ignore the negative energy. The situation becomes magnified and aggravated when neither is able to be honest and assertive with the other. They are incapable of expressing their true feelings appropriately or responsibly. Plus, the son-in-law and grandchildren are now exposed to the effects of an unhealthy relationship.

One Resolution—the ABC Method

According to Lange and Jakobowski (1976), Ellis's ABC Method is a way to help daughters like N restructure the self-talk that creates such situations and feelings of fear, anxiety, frustration, and guilt. Similar to the concept of perceptual shift, a mental shift can give our computer-like brain a message that allows us to bypass emotional reactions and restructure our thinking.

The ABC method is easily illustrated by placing the letters A, B, and C across a board or flip chart as the titles of three columns. (A) represents the *activating* event, (B) represents the thoughts and *belief system*, and (C) represents the *consequence* or bad feelings of guilt, fear, hurt, or anger.

To process the previous vignette, ask the group to fill in the columns. Start with (C). What is the consequence, or N's bad feeling? Let's say the students said it was *guilt*. Now move to (A). What caused the guilt? Answer, mother living alone so far away. Question, was that really the cause? Go to (B). No, it was N's belief, her perception that she had to take care of her mother. When visually depicted, the impact of the message is more potent. Here the students can see that it was how N perceived and interpreted the situation that triggered the emotional decision.

What we tell ourselves, what we believe, how we label that belief, and what the event means to our personal systems of valuing and operating create how we respond and make our own problems, not the event itself.

If N had shifted her self-talk, the guilt feelings would have disappeared and the "I'm Only Trying To Help" game would have stopped. Honesty and assertiveness would have been possible. N might have been able to identify her true feelings, perceive her mother's need for control, and say,

"Mother, I'm concerned about your being by yourself and so far away from us. I also know it would not be best for either you or me to have you come and live with us, but if you want, I'm willing to help you move to an apartment or retirement home near us."

N is now clear on what she is willing to do, has removed the guilt feelings, and has expressed her decision appropriately and responsibly. Refusal to play the game has started.

Behavioral Rehearsal and Role Playing

Now that N has cleared her thinking and knows exactly what she wants to say and do, the next step is behavioral rehearsal or role play. Essentially, it is N setting up the scenario, selecting her protagonist (mother), explaining what is wanted, and role playing the situation. Before you start, however, make certain N's thinking is still clear. Without such clarity, the role play and follow-up practice are ineffective. Having a trained coach to facilitate this process is therefore helpful, because he or she can abort the rehearsal if the thinking is convoluted and then lead the assertor back through the cognitive restructuring process.

Coaching

As the workshop facilitator, you will probably have to be the coach in the beginning, the person who monitors and guides the process, as well as demonstrate the assertive skills required. Broken down into specific steps, the role play process is as follows:

1. N establishes the scene and players involved.
2. N chooses a protagonist (P) whom she thinks can mimic her mother's mannerisms, words, and attitude.
3. N then tells P how and what her mother would likely say and do, being as specific as possible.
4. N then states clearly what she wants to say to P. (N may need to write this down and repeat it first.)
5. The scene opens with a greeting and short buildup to the desired confrontation. N's brief, practiced, and succinct statement follows, with P (or mother) agreeing with N's assertion to make it initially easy.
6. Coach stops the interaction and asks N to say what she liked about what she did. (Be persistent here, nothing negative at this point. Also, focus in on the nonverbals: space, posture, movement, facial expressions, eyes, tone of voice, pauses, and speed.)
7. When N is through with her self-assessment, P and finally the group do the same without repeating what N said. (Keep the class focused on the positive, for example, "I liked the way you . . . " This is critical in the initial phases of building N's self-confidence.)
8. Coach now asks N if there is anything she would do differently next time. N responds, as do P and the group. (Careful monitoring is required here.)
9. The whole process is now repeated at least three times, escalating the negativity each time until N is self-assured and her responses are automatic.
10. End with a commitment from N to report back to the group the following week, or as soon as feasible, the results of her confrontation with her mother.

Note. Feedback from the observers here is essential to the learning process because it sharpens their ability to pick up on the nonverbals, often the unconscious triggers to a game.

Practice, Practice, Practice

Paramount to becoming assertive is practice and then more practice. This means drilling over and over and over again, until old patterns are turned into new responses that are automatic and effective the minute the next toxic attack occurs. It means that the new responses forcefully but quietly communicate "I mean what I say." It means, be patient with yourself. It takes time to get the phraseology and the nonverbal messages congruent, time to make certain the words and the body language are being interpreted accurately.

To facilitate the practice of confrontation in love, divide the remaining class participants into triads (assertor, protagonist, and coach) as soon as the behavioral rehearsal demonstration with N is completed. Ask the triads to go through the same role play steps as the demonstration until they are comfortable with the process.

Initially, a simulated scenario on which all class members work simultaneously can be quite effective. It allows the students to clarify any uncertainties, to internalize the steps, and to compare the differences in how each triad handles the situation. After that, it is best to move to personal situations, and the formation of support triads for ongoing practice outside of the class or workshop. (An easy scenario for the initial attempt will be offered.)

Just make certain that the students first check their motives for confronting a toxic ager. It is essential that these motives represent an authentic attempt, expressed in love, to clear the air and establish honest, open communication, not to put their parent or client down, tell them off, or change them into what the students want.

A Simulated Scenario for Service Providers

If the workshop or class is made up of service providers, the following scenario might be helpful. You, as a social worker or director are confronting, for the fifth time, a 77-year-old toxic regular (X) at a senior center. X is known to complain incessantly about her troubles and always in a loud, high-pitched, harsh voice that everyone in the building can hear. No matter what subject you try to focus on, there is a detour into endless explanations of similar incidents in her younger days, plus tales of how cruel people have been to her, tales repeated at each encounter *ad nauseum.* There is no indication X is listening to anything you say. In every attempt you make to question, confront, or control the interaction, X attacks with a look of defensive fear and terror in her eyes, a facial wince, a toss of her head, and then back to the incessant, disruptive complaints that have nothing to do with what you were attempting to get her to focus on.

Role Play

For the best effect, and fun, have a few students prepared in advance to role play the scene initially. This adds a dramatic stage setting for all who are participating. Triads are then formed for the behavioral rehearsal practice. Roles are chosen. Decisions are made as to what the center director or social worker wants to accomplish and precisely how he or she will assertively say it to X. Role-play steps are then practiced, and assessment occurs. Feedback follows from each triad, explaining how they assertively solved the situation and what they learned, followed by summary processing in the large group.

Another fun alternative for the exercise is to have each triad act out their assertive solution and then proceed to large group processing. Also consider videotaping for instant feedback and self-evaluation and group evaluation.

Summary

Despite the fact that this chapter concentrates on strategies and techniques, caution is advised in using them only as supplementary tools or springboards for your own creativity in stimulating a learning exercise. Acknowledge first, however, that you are your greatest asset. Your being, your caring presence, starts the healing process.

Because the basic assumption of this book is that toxics can only heal themselves and therefore cannot be fixed, the approach here is to interrupt the toxic loop and game systems that reinforce their toxicity. This means essentially that the role of the therapist is changed to that of the educator, teaching primarily adult children of toxic agers, especially those who are gerontology professionals, how to break the co-Victim cycle. It means teaching service providers what to expect and how to set limits, work with the adult children, and not hook into the games. It means teaching early-stage toxics who recognize and own their toxicity and want desperately to change, as well as older adults who fear toxicity and are seeking to prevent it. It means coordinating the efforts of all involved with toxics to interrupt and stop the game cycle.

In my experience, the best approach is a combined workshop and support group format. Details are provided on how to design the contents and the structure and facilitate these groups based on my ACTA (Adult Children of Toxic Agers) workshop and support group model. Strategies also include structured interventions, referral resources, exercises, and case examples of ineffective negative coping.

Techniques include perceptual shift, the goodbye letter, vignettes, and case scenarios on how to identify and stop games, as well as how to facilitate the key aspects of Responsible Assertion Training: cognitive restructuring, behavioral rehearsal, coaching, and Ellis's ABC method.

Part V

Is Toxicity Preventable? Is Healing Possible?

Try to apply seriously what I have told you, not that you might escape suffering—nobody can escape it—but that you may avoid the worst—blind suffering.

—Author unknown

Chapter 13

Self-Help and Prevention

Over and over again the plea is heard!

"I don't want to be like that!"

It is a proclamation that seethes with agony and pained memories, a giveaway that the proclaimer is the son or daughter of a toxic ager. It is a call for help from adult children, themselves older adults, who unconsciously sense they too are becoming toxic. It is an inner fear, a conviction that they are drowning, hopelessly sinking in frustration, guilt, and despair . . .

and they are.

But they need not be. No one wants to be toxic. No one wants to be consumed by a psychological poison that eats away inside, out of our awareness. Although toxic tendencies may be genetic, the Victim consciousness of toxicity is learned. Therefore, it can be interrupted. If recognized early, the patterns can be broken. Further deterioration can be prevented. Even reversal is possible. It just is not easy. It means persistent effort. It takes individual determination, motivation, energy, practice, and support. It takes an awakening to the syndrome, a public acceptance of its reality, and an acknowledgment that toxicity is not a sin. It takes a perceptual shift.

Toxicity in agers is an anomaly,* an anomaly that takes a lifetime of conditioned responses to build. It cannot be fixed, but the behavioral patterns displayed can be modified, possibly even dismantled, albeit slowly, piece by piece.

Real change, however, means awakening to the self-deceit, the illusions, with which we all live. It means acknowledging the symptoms. It means being accountable to a different belief system, a different perceptual response pattern, a different attention to values, a different modeling of behavior, a different understanding of truth, a different sense of Self, and a different grasp and application of love: unconditional love. It means living that which most of us now only profess. If we can live it, however, toxicity can be prevented.

Candidates for Self-Help

Adult children of toxic agers (including professionals) are not the only ones who are candidates for self-help. Others might include older adults who fear becoming toxic and want to prevent it from developing, who realize they are toxic prone and want to break the cycle, or who already recognize some symptoms of toxicity in themselves and are determined to reverse the trend. All are promising aspirants for self-help.

Some agers, however, would find the journey into wholeness too difficult, particularly those in the early stages of grief and those who are brain damaged, mentally ill, clinically or chronically depressed, or in the advanced stages of toxicity, alcoholism, or some other mental or emotional impairment.

Self-Help Tips

For those of you who are ready and motivated, there are many ways to help yourself. First, however, a reminder. It may take months of watchful self-discipline, plus a determination and willingness to experiment with the variety of possibilities available until you find the one(s) that fit your personality type.

In order to make some sense out of the various self-help approaches offered, they have been arranged in different categories consisting of self-nourishment, stress management, stress reduction, support groups, and special programs, all of which result in some form of perceptual shift. Case stories will help to illustrate the subjects whenever possible. The key is to recognize that the real self-help work is within, discovering what works for you and then doing it—daily.

Self-Nourishment and Warm Fuzzies

Self-nourishing people simply do not become toxic. They know they are responsible for taking care of themselves. They know how to give themselves positive strokes, to love and protect themselves, and to express their feelings honestly and appropriately. If toxic prone, they know they must be vigilant in removing any fears or negativity that block their self-love in order to prevent the deep-seated anger and pain of toxicity from invading.

They also know that self-nourishment, or "warm fuzzies," must become a mandatory routine, scheduled "right off the top" until it becomes habitual and automatic, usually a period of 3 months. Yes, it is a challenge.

Self-Affirmations

Self-affirmations are a form of uplifting positive strokes that will help you feel good about yourself. The best way to practice self-affirmations is to say them at least three times a day to start with, or every hour, or even every 5 minutes if possible. Frequent repetition blocks out the negative thoughts and is useful in reducing distress, anxiety, fear, and guilt, and is helpful in getting you to sleep.

To attain the most benefit, however, it is important to keep all affirmations positive and in the first person, present tense, usually starting with the words, "I am." Avoid all negative terms such as not, don't, won't, and never—because the computer-like brain will input them as disaffirmations. After saying the affirmation, begin to act "as if" the words are true, even though you may not believe them at first. They are not gimmicks or egotism unless you perceive them as such. Anytime you do something new and different or contrary to your usual patterns, it may feel peculiar, silly, and even uncomfortable at first. Just hang in, and trust the process.

Some examples of self-affirmations are as follows:

I am lovable, capable, esteemed, caring.

I am wonderful, responsible, worthy, loving.

I am doing what is best for all of us.

Within me are all the resources I need.

I am OK. I am good. I am valued.

Self-affirmations also help us to feel our personal power, to know that "in charge" sense of potency, and to awaken us to the realization that we do not need to depend on others to give us the nurturance we need, nor is it wise. Some people may insist on meeting our needs, often an unhealthy form of manipulative control. Others are capable of meeting our needs but forget to do it or do not want the bother. Be wary of both types. No one can know what we need unless we tell them (see the section on Target Strokes later), since no one can read our minds. Those close to us will think they know what we need, but invariably it is a projection. We get what *they* think we need, not what *we* need.

Other Warm Fuzzies

Mirror Talk

Each morning, when you first get up, look in the mirror (before shaving, combing your hair, or putting on your makeup) and say with gusto, "I love you."

At first it will feel weird. Several of my students even shut the door so no one would see or hear them. Whatever works is OK. Just do it. The point is to be able to look beyond the surface and see the love and beauty that is deep inside. When you can, relish adding other words like, "You're terrific!"

Love Notes

Write yourself love notes or letters, full of positive declarations, then mail them. Or put a self-affirmation on your refrigerator, mirror, or car dashboard. Make a tape and play it over and over as you are driving. Just be creative.

Quiet Time

"Make" at least 20 to 30 minutes a day available (start with 5 minutes if that is all you can get) for you to go within, to breathe deeply and just sit, meditate, reflect, think, read, write, listen to music, pray, write in your journal, or whatever works for you. This is your time to center, to spiritually focus, to listen to that Inner Voice, and to seek some inner peace. It is sacred time. Honor it and yourself.

Dance Time

This one I discovered just last summer while rewriting this book. It is especially great if you have stereophonic surround sound. Select your favorite music (for me it is Big Band). Turn it up loud, with full bass, close your eyes, and dance to the beat. Guided by your heart, just let your body flow with whatever comes. I guarantee, you will forget everything. Even if it is for only 5 minutes, you will feel better and be reenergized.

Personal "Me Time"

Me Time is different from Quiet Time. The focus here is on a special time, a break in your daily routine just for you, to do whatever you want because you are important. The key is that it cannot be anything you *have* to do. Start with 5 minutes a day and work up to 60 minutes, if possible. It could be a time to have a cup of coffee, to call a friend, or to read your favorite book. It could be time for stretching and exercising such as yoga, tai chi, walking, aerobics, tennis, swimming, bicycling, or going to the spa. It could be time for gardening; taking a class; working on a fun project, hobby, or arts and crafts; or hiring a sitter so you can give some volunteer service to your community or church.

Me Time could be arranging for your spouse or friends to take the kids or grandma to the park so you can soak in a hot bubble bath with soft music. It could be getting a respite sitter to care for Dad so you can go shopping or to the beach or take a hike in the woods. It is going to your bedroom, or a quiet spot, the minute you get home from work, shutting the door, and reading for 30 minutes to defuse a rough day at the office. Just do not forget the "Do Not Disturb" sign! (Of course, this needs to be a prearranged contract established for that special occasion when you are exhausted and vulnerable and want to prevent hooking into toxic games such as Poor Me, Uproar, and Let's You and Him Fight.)

Whatever the Me Time, the ideas are limited only by your own imagination and creativity. Do whatever it takes to slow the mind and give you a feeling of joy and inner peace, as long as it is appropriate to the situation and does not infringe on the rights and considerations of others. All it takes is for you to structure the time into your daily or weekly schedule, then maintain it with religious fervor for at least a 3-month commitment. The outcome is worth it.

Just remember, do not get too smug about how smart you are for doing this for yourself. It also does wonders for everyone who has to live and work with you.

Target Strokes

As might be suspected from the title, target strokes are a concept from TA and another way of getting nurturance, recognition, and love. Although also considered positive strokes or warm fuzzies, target strokes are specific and unique. They are personalized ways to get the nourishment we either forget or are unable to give to ourselves if we are in a negative space. With target strokes, tensions are relieved, things are put back into perspective, and a warm feeling surges throughout the body. We feel good inside because we know someone cared enough to make the effort to give us what we needed when we needed it.

To be effective, target strokes must be prearranged. To do this, a verbal contract is made with someone you see almost daily (coworkers often work better than family) and can trust to carry out your request. The first step is to be clear on the kind of target stroke you want or need, to assess its appropriateness for either a public or a private environment, and then to find and ask the person if he or she is willing to carry out the arrangement. If the answer is yes, describe to the person, in precise detail, the *exact* kind of warm fuzzy you want when he or she sees signs that you have not been nurturing or taking care of yourself.

Usually these signs of self-nurturing neglect are clear. They will consist of an energy drop, moodiness, withdrawal, irritability, spitefulness, restlessness, depression, or any other atypical negative behavior. These signs mean you have not given yourself the affirmations you need to sustain your self-love, nor have you asked for the strokes needed to bring yourself back up. When a coworker, friend, or family member notices your signs of personal neglect, his or her role is to give you (without a word) your exact prearranged target stroke as quickly as possible.

By nature, these individualized target strokes vary widely. For a work environment desired strokes might be a back rub, a hug, a note saying what a terrific job you are doing, bringing you your favorite tea or coffee, or covering for you while you take a break. For the personal or home area the target stroke might be (in addition to the above) a more intimate touch or holding, a foot or body massage, a couple of hours of respite, a night out, a love note on the pillow, a walk in the park, doing the dishes, cleaning the house, taking care of the kids for a few hours, some special Me Time, or simply the words "I love you," whispered in your ear with a warm hug.

Whatever is chosen, the warm fuzzy target stroke must be something both the receiver and the giver agree to target in order to be effective. The key is doing *exactly* what the receiver requested, at the right time, and in the right way.

Scenario

One descriptive example of this process is a story I tell often. Several years ago I was conducting a TA staff development workshop for a social service agency. As part of the training I had the staff share their target strokes with their coworkers. One caseworker told the group her target stroke was peanut butter. She felt it was weird, but she had a real passion for it. Everyone giggled, and we went on. The following week, however, I was met at the door with a loud exclamation, "It works! It works!"

It seems that this seasoned professional had come into the office one day shortly after our workshop very upset about something that had happened at home. In a way unlike her usual self, she promptly proceeded to unprofessionally spew her negativity and problems onto everyone within earshot—clients, coworkers, volunteers, even the public. This lasted past lunch and into the afternoon. Everyone gave her a wide berth. When she returned from her afternoon break, however, there on her desk sat a huge jar of peanut butter. The impact was sudden and strong. The negative energy seemed to literally evaporate. Feeling loved again, she returned to her usual caring self. Someone had remembered and cared enough to give her her target stroke.

The problems this professional was experiencing at home had not gone away. The peanut butter, however, was the jolting shift that boosted her spirits and restored enough self-esteem to enable her to cope with her situation, as well as place it back where it belonged: at home.

Translate this scenario into your own self-help goal and ask yourself these questions. What kind of support system do I have when things are overwhelming and I am not taking care of myself? What is my target stroke? Whom have I told? Do I have a commitment that they will follow through when I need them?

Stress Management

Manage stress? Why? Stress is normal. It is part of life. It is the energy stimulant that often moves us to action. It helps us feel alive, that is, until it gets out of balance, beyond management, and excessive. Then stress is trouble. Then it becomes distress. Then, we manage it.

Stress management is a learned skill. It is also a basic concept for self-helpers. Through effective management, you can recognize and establish your own level of optimal personal stress and develop your own program of wellness practices and holistic health (explained in more detail in the last chapter). With these practices you can maintain a self-nourishing system that can prevent social, emotional, physical, mental, and spiritual toxicity, as well as help to heal deep toxic scars.

Subjective Units of Discomfort Scale—
Measuring Optimal Stress Levels

The Subjective Units of Discomfort Scale (*SUDS*) is actually an internal stress management scale measuring the degree of distress and anxiety (Figure 13.1). The range is from 0 to 100. At 0 we are catatonic, at 100 we have exploded; 50 is the average level, but few people are at that point. The optimal levels of stress vary widely according to each individual. Some of us are racehorses and operate at a high stress pace, with the optimal level at about

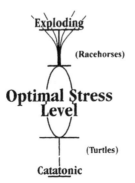

FIGURE 13.1   SUDS.

75. Others are turtles and work best at a slower stress pace, with the optimal level around 25.

Identifying Your SUDS Level

The task for each of you is to ignore what others say, determine your own unique and most comfortable level of energy, honor your red flag signals, and be alert for imbalance and excesses. Then monitor your SUDS level daily, conscientiously maintaining it at your optimal level. If you have either too much or too little stress, it is doubtful you will have the stamina to withstand a toxic's attack. Distress is painful at either end of the continuum.

Excessive stress creates "burnout" or "blowout" and can be recognized by high blood pressure, fast pulse, sweaty hands, flushed face, nervous stomach, irritability, compulsiveness, impatience, or whatever your response pattern may be. Too little stress creates "rust out" and can be recognized by lethargy, dullness, depression, lack of energy, apathy, hopelessness, indifference, and withdrawal. Both extremes are serious.

Stress proliferation is common and relentless if we do not own and recognize our own stressors and reorder our energy and priorities accordingly. A primary stressor, such as an external situation with which you must deal, may not be the major problem. Much depends on your own internal (intrapsychic) condition and state of mind, which often generates the debilitating secondary stressors. These stressors, according to Aneshensel, Pearlin, Mullan, Zarit, and Whitlatch (1995) in their longitudinal study of caregivers, can cause a depressive secondary role strain and a loss of self and role overload from the intrapsychic strain. As defined by these researchers, stressors are "conditions, experiences, and activities that are problematic for people, threatening to them, thwarting their efforts, fatiguing them, and defeating their dreams" (1995, p. 69).

A few strategies for reducing these stressors and maintaining your SUDS at the optimal level follow. Actually, any of the other suggestions found in this chapter and the Wellness Practices in the next chapter can be applied if you find them helpful.

Meditation

Meditation is one of those necessities for the "racehorses" (working care providers?) who dash around all day, never take a breather, never sit still, and do not know the meaning of the word "relax," even if they could. Meditation is usually a disciplined "practice" of 20 minutes or more a day that has a high priority in the day's agenda. Ideally, it becomes a way of life, a way to empty conscious thought and be open to an inner spiritual peace.

There are many varieties of meditation, from the pure receptiveness of Zen sitting to the calming movements of tai chi and the postures of yoga; the absorption of poetry, art, music, or nature; contemplative walking; the rapture of a sunset; the formal structure of Transcendental Meditation (TM). Many books, articles, workshops, training programs, and meditation groups are available to teach the particulars of each practice. All require commitment and self-discipline.

The kind of meditation you choose depends upon your own personal preference, personality type or temperament, and culture or style of living. There is no best way. Experiment until you find the form that works for you. Individuals who "go inside" easily or readily slip into daydreaming or reflection, probably will profit more from an active type of meditation. Individuals who are very active will likewise usually gain more from an inward, contemplative meditation. That is not always true, however. Check them out, then choose the form that you are most comfortable with.

The critical element in meditation is that you *make* the time to meditate. The easiest way is simply to structure it into your daily schedule until it becomes a habit. For professionals who work with difficult, emotionally taxing situations or caregivers and adult children of toxic agers, the quieting of a daily routine of meditation practice is amazingly sustaining, and effective stress management.

Relaxation Response

If you do not have time to meditate, practice the relaxation response. It takes only 5 minutes once a day. It not only helps manage stress but also is effective as a coping strategy, particularly if also practiced as a quieting process just before each encounter with a toxic ager.

The relaxation response was developed and perfected by Herbert Benson, M.D., over many years of treating patients in his holistic health clinic. Even today Benson continues to promote the power of the mind and body to work together as a unified system of healing and interconnecting communication.

The first step in practicing the relaxation response is to find a quiet comfortable place. After settling down, take three deep breaths. Then choose a mantra, a key word, or a meaningful phrase to say to yourself over and over for 3 to 5 minutes until you feel peaceful and serene inside. The phrase could be your favorite scripture, a saying, or even a nonsensical term such as "one" or "om" or anything to force concentration on something other than the tension in your body or the chatter in your head. Your body will respond with reduced metabolism, heart rate, and blood pressure. Any frustration or internal chatter in your mind will generally settle, often into a calmness that enables you to face more stressors.

Self-Talk

Although similar to self-affirmations, self-talk is focused specifically on maintaining positive thinking and changing negative inner tapes through cognitive restructuring. It is similar to "psyching yourself up" before a stressful event. It is saying to yourself as you anticipate a visit with an advanced toxic client or parent,

I am clear in what I need and want

I am in control of the situation

I am setting the boundaries

I am staying in charge

I am not responsible for making her happy

I accept her as she is

She can say anything; I am free from her games

Self-talk, like affirmations, is fed into the hypothalamus control center in the brain, which in turn sends the message to the rest of the body. Because it is a feedback network, if the words are positive, the system signals a confirmation that all is OK. The more frequently messages are sent, the more established becomes the sense of being OK. It is similar to a computer system. If we fill it with garbage, we will get garbage out. If I'm telling myself that

I'm capable

I can handle this

I'll make it

I'm on top of the situation

the body and mind will respond accordingly. If I'm telling myself

No one understands

I can't please her

I can't go on

It's hopeless

the body systems respond in kind.

Together, these basic systems (nervous, circulatory, digestive, respiratory, and elimination) methodically carry out the messages given to them. No questions asked. The computer-like brain has no way of discriminating whether a message is negative or positive, made up or actual. It simply receives and sends whatever it is fed. If it gets negativity or garbage, then garbage is circulated. The trouble is, garbage soon begins to deteriorate, causing the body and mind to react. It is a form of negative programming we all experience, especially toxics, as we talk ourselves into all forms of mental, emotional, and physical "dis-ease."

Take a look at your own self-talk. Then, as you assess it ask yourself

1. Do I really know what I tell myself everyday?
2. If it's negative, do I want it to control my life?
3. Do I want the consequences?
4. What am I going to do about it?

Reversing Negative Self-Talk

There are several ways to reverse negative self-talk. First, we need to identify what it is we tell ourselves. The following is a format I found helpful with my students. Using a large sheet of paper lengthwise, divide it into four perpendicular columns labeled: Date/Time, Trigger, Negative Thought, and Positive Thought. For the next 2 weeks, keeping the write-ups as brief and succinct as possible, record the date, time, and situation when the negative thought(s) occur. Then immediately change the undermining statement into a positive one. This last step is the most critical. First, it forces you to shift your perception. Second, the intensive focus on the negative tends to ignite depressive feelings; it is therefore imperative that you complete the last column and make it positive.

At the end of each week, review what you have written. Look for patterns, what or who triggered the negative thought, the feelings associated, and what difference the shift to the positive made. Then note what you uncovered or learned. Report this back to a prearranged support person and talk about it for further clarification. If faithfully undertaken and processed, this can be a revealing exercise.

Journaling

Journaling is another powerful tool for self-nourishment. Numerous how-to books and workshops exist on the process. Choose the process that fits you, then develop your own system. For the best results, give it a consistent 3 months' trial, writing in it daily or as the need arises. Journaling is not a diary or a log. Instead, it provides a private opportunity for you to vent your feelings and to express, recognize, own, and bring whatever might be festering inside into conscious awareness, enabling you to deal with it or let it go. Keep the journal focused on feelings (especially anger, frustration, guilt, and hopelessness). Examine your perceptions and write affirmations or even dialogue with your toxic ager or your anger, your pain, even your higher Self. Be creative.

Dialoguing

Because dialoguing is a special aspect of journaling, I want to give it more attention. Before you begin, it works best to allow yourself some time to get quiet or centered. Soft music is helpful. Find a private place and take the phone off the hook at a time when there will be no interruptions. Have a notebook and pen ready and, with eyes half shut, start by asking who or whatever you are dialoguing with a question. Then wait. The answer will come from an inner voice, a sense, image, or thought. Write it down as it comes. No censoring or interpreting. Follow with other questions, letting the dialogue flow. Continue until you feel complete. Results can be surprising, nourishing, releasing, or provocative. Problems can be resolved, emotions calmed, and solutions reached.

Stress Reduction

Stress reduction is different from stress management. Instead of directing and controlling stress, stress reduction is primarily for coping with stress and reducing the strain. Usually accomplished through skills and techniques, it enables you to deal with immediate problems, not prevent them. Coping skills are imperative when contending with difficult situations in life. They save the moment. They do not, however, change anything or prevent a toxic flare-up from occurring in the first place. They are a must, however, for dealing with toxic agers. Some stress reduction skills are discussed in what follows.

Deep Breathing

Deep breathing is the easiest and perhaps the most effective technique for coping with distress situations. It can be practiced anywhere, anytime, in the office with a belligerent client, during a conflict, when you are feeling overwhelmed, or your parent is whining and complaining. Three deep breaths will force enough oxygen to the brain to enable you to think clearly and calm yourself down.

There are some specific steps for deep breathing. They are as follows:

1. Just remembering to do it.
2. Close your eyes (optional) and concentrate on your breathing.
3. Take a deep breath that goes all the way down into your extended abdomen and (like a wave) back up to the chest.
4. Breathe in to the count of four, hold it for the count of eight, then breathe out to the count of twelve. This automatically slows things down.
5. Once the rhythm is natural and the situation permits, you may substitute any phrase that works for you, such as *I am* as you breathe in and *relaxed* as you breathe out, or *I am love . . . manifesting,* or *I am . . . strong,* or *I am in . . . control,* or *understanding,* or *patient.*

Deep breathing always helps if the SUDS level is excessive. Reason? When we are in anticipation or under stress, we almost forget to breathe. It becomes so shallow, the brain does not get the nourishment it needs. Like the rest of our body, when our brain is undernourished, it sends distress signals throughout the nervous system. Our SUDS level automatically rises. Problem solving and objective thinking are lowered. If we are smart, it is the time to stay away from toxics until our stress-reduction practice brings us back to our optimal level of functioning.

Assertive Skills

Time Out

In addition to being a coping technique, as mentioned in chapter 11 (on p. 204), Time Out is an effective tool to reduce conflict and excess SUDS levels, essential for both professionals and lay people in keeping their mental and emotional health in balance when coping with toxic agers.

Whenever you sense your SUDS level is going beyond your optimal point and you are losing control, proclaim a Time Out. This is especially critical in game playing, when you slide into your Child ego state and are no longer functioning in your objective, rational Adult state. As soon as you catch the shift into your Child, interrupt the other game player, look him or her square in the eye, and state assertively that you need some Time Out and will be back in 10 or 15 minutes. Then, leave before you get rehooked into the game. Just be sure you return as stated.

Stroke and Stand

Helpful when you want a toxic to hear you, Stroke and Stand is a positive statement or compliment that states clearly and firmly what you intend or want. For example,

Dad, you've been very good to me in the past and I appreciate that. However, I will no longer put up with your controls and demands. From here on I will make my own decisions.

Broken Record

Broken Record is essentially a way to repeat or rephrase a statement over and over until the other person recognizes you mean what you say and gives up. Caution: just use judgment on how far you push.

Mother, I am not able to visit you every day. I will call daily to see how you are, but my visits will be limited to three or four times a week.

Mother responds with her whiny Poor Me. Firmly, and without recognizing her lamenting, repeat the statement. Do not add anything. In fact, if mother seems to refuse to hear you, shorten your sentence with each repeat. If needed, reword it slightly, making it more emphatic until she realizes you will not be there every day. If she escalates after three repeats, take a Time Out and return to repeat your assertion. Just be sure that in the end you follow through and do what you said you would.

Fogging

Similar to TA's game stopper of giving an unexpected answer, Fogging's purpose is to give an inane response that implies you agree with what was said but commits you to nothing. For example, Mother goes on one of her tirades, calling you a selfish, uncaring, thoughtless daughter. You respond with something like

> Yes, mother, it may appear that way. Sometimes I do come across as thoughtless, uncaring, and selfish.

Make your statement short and quick, then change immediately to another subject. Again, it is another way to avoid the game hook. In all cases, use appropriate and effective body language. Remember, it takes practice.

I Messages

A must if you want direct and honest communication, I Messages are especially vital in a long-term relationship with an elderly toxic spouse. An example of this is

> Martha, I care about you and want what is best for both of us, but I will not violate who I am. That means I am standing firm in loving and being myself, and that will not always please you.

Often, most of us start a statement with "You" or "Why," only to discover the other person immediately becomes defensive. I messages avoid that hook, and open the door for honest, game-free interaction.

Game Stopping

If you find yourself in a second- or third-*degree* psychological game and manage to stop it, I guarantee your stress will be reduced.

Remember the signs of a game: (1) it takes two to play, (2) both players are subconsciously conditioned to know the rules, (3) both are unaware that they are playing unless they recognize the bad-feeling *payoff* at the end of the game, (4) there is an ulterior hidden agenda, and (5) the game will go on indefinitely until someone chooses not to play. That someone is the Nurturing Parent in you who takes control and says "stop" to the inner Child who loves to play. If the transaction is then shifted to the Adult ego state, the game is permanently stopped. If you stay in your Adult, there are no more games, no more dishonesty. It is that simple. The Adult in you does not play games (Berne, 1964).

The key to game-stopping is to discover what is hooking your Child. The first step is to recognize the bad-feeling payoff after a game and then see if you can trace your response back to what it was that triggered the initial hook. For instance, when did your body language shift into the Child ego state? Check for nonverbal clues; there will be visible changes in your tone of voice, body posture, movements, and facial expressions. Once you uncover the game trigger you can avoid the hook the next time by simply choosing to stay in your Adult. No one is forced to play a game. The consequences and responsibility are yours if you decide to continue playing.

Support Networks and Groups

In the early 1980s, the California Department of Mental Health conducted a 5-year research program to discover the key ingredient for the development of good mental and emotional health. The answer they found was surprising. It was simply, supportive friends, groups, and networks. It seemed too simple. No fancy psychological training or treatment, just people; people who not only care about and understand each other's situation, but also feel and share each other's pain; people who support and trust each other; people who show their love, are always there for each other, and become true friends. It is possible, and it heals.

Personal Story

Growing up in a toxic family of fearful, frightened, and demeaning people, H, an ex-student of mine, never learned to love or esteem herself. She lived with anxiety and emotional abuse that resulted in her constantly discounting herself. Nothing she did was good enough. Mother was unpleasable. It seems that the only way mother knew how to assuage her deep-seated fears was to control.

Marriage to a university professor was H's escape, she thought. Four children were born and raised while H attempted to cope with her spouse's growing alcoholism and toxicity. With no sense of personal power or self-esteem, H put up with physical, as well as emotional, abuse. Depressed, heavily medicated, and hospitalized from his assaults she finally realized she did not have to accept the abuse. She took the children and moved across the country, as far away as she could get.

Forced now to make it on her own, H found inner resources she never believed she had. She attended Al-Anon, AA meetings, and the 12-Step Program and found people who cared. She went often. The positive feedback helped. She sought some grants and reentered college, determined to make something of herself. Six years of counseling, working part time, scholarships, assertion and self-esteem building classes, Dale Carnegie training, ongoing support groups, plus the demands of school helped her begin to believe in herself. With every opportunity, she pushed herself to take on a new challenge, climaxing with her LCSW, a career in the gerontology field, and speaking engagements to encourage other reentry students and victims of abuse. All possible, says H, because people cared, had faith in her, gave her reliable steady support, and helped her find herself.

At this writing, H works with toxic agers almost daily and may be overheard proclaiming to them, "You can be as toxic as you want. I'm still going to do it, because I care about you." Audiences will hear,

"People need love the most when they deserve it the least."

Special Programs

Special self-help programs and teachings are profuse today, available to anyone seeking help. The key is to go out and find the ones in which you are comfortable. H did.

Many self-help programs are designed to enable you to discover clarity and truth and resolve difficult situations and relationships. One such teaching is an exercise developed by Byron Katie in Barstow, California. She calls it "The Work." I'm presenting it here because I believe it is particularly applicable to older adults who fear they might become toxic, early stage toxics who want to change, or any adult child with a difficult parent–child relationship, especially those who happen to also be professionals in the gerontology field. As you examine The Work, notice the pervasiveness of the perceptual shift philosophy throughout.

The Work

The little booklet that explains The Work and is distributed by Katie in her workshops is entitled *What to Do When Nothing Works* (Katie, 1996). With Katie's permission, the six steps to her process are described. Read the directions. Then, as conscientiously as possible, complete your responses from the point of view of an angry, hurt, sad, or frightened 3- or 4-year old. This is critical to the success of your work. Do not try to be realistic or analyze anything, just point your finger and judge whomever, or whatever, you feel is responsible for your pain. Write anything that comes up in response to the statements. No thinking. Be as petty, child-like, and honest as possible, just follow the instructions precisely. A sample is placed within the brackets.

1. Write about a situation beginning with
   I don't like (name) _____ **because he/she** _____ (describe what he/she did to you) or
   I am angry at or saddened by (name) _____ [*mother*] **because** _____ [*she never listens to me. She's selfish. She makes me feel bad* _____].
2. **I want (name)** _____ **to** [*hear me*] _____.
   List the things you want (name) to do, be, think, or feel in this situation.
3. **(Name)** _____ **shouldn't or should** [*care about me*].
   List the things that (name) _____ should or shouldn't do, be, think, or feel in this situation.

4. **(Name)** _____ **is** [*not nice. She's mean.*] _____.
   List the things (name) _____ is in this situation.

5. **I need (name)** _____ **to** [*love me*] _____.
   List the things that (name) _____ might give you or could do in order for you to be happy in this situation. Judge only him or her and not yourself.

6. **I am not willing to or I won't ever** [*be like her*] _____.
   Here list the things that you refuse to do or that you think you will never do again.

Exercise Key

Once you have completed the written portion, take time to go within (and tap into the guidance of your Adult and Nurturing Parent ego states) and get in touch with your own Truths. Although this can be undertaken by yourself, the best effect is usually with a guide or friend.

1. Looking at your original answer, read your situation aloud. Then stop and be still. Read it again and ask yourself, is it true? Did **(name)** _____ do it? Is she or he really _____? Can I know that, honestly?
   Now reverse each sentence and read, **I don't like me because** [*I'm selfish*] _____ or **I am angry at me because** [*I don't listen to me; I make me feel bad*] _____.
   Which statement is the most truthful, the original or your reversal? Know that pointed fingers are considered to be a mirror reflection of ourselves.

2. Read each statement again aloud. Go inside. Be still. Ask yourself, is it true? What is the payoff for holding that belief? What is in it for me? Who would I be without this belief? Again, reverse each statement to, **I want me to** [*hear*] _____. Then add, **I want me to** [*hear me*] _____. Is that true? Practice here keeping your mind on your own business.

3. Read your list aloud. Go within. Be still. Then read again. Ask yourself, can I know that really? What is in it for me to have that thought? Should **(name)** _____ have to change his or her life for my sake? Who would I be without that

belief?

Now reverse it to **I (shouldn't) or should** [*care about me*] _____ **when I think that** [*mother*] _____ **should** [*care about me*] _____. This reversal reveals a self-prescription. Follow through on it.

4. With each question, continue the same pattern. Always ask yourself with each statement, is it true? Can I know that? What is my reward for holding on to this belief? What would I be without it? If there is no way out, just call it "hopeless" and go on.

 Again reverse each statement saying, for example, **I am** [*not nice*] _____, **and I am** [*mean*] _____ **when I see** [*mother*] _____ **as** [*mean*] _____ **to me**.

 Is this where your anger or hurt really comes from? Was it what he or she did or your judgments (projections) about it that really hurt? Stay in your own business.

5. Again, repeat your statement, and so on, and ask yourself, is it true? Can I know that? What is the payoff for holding on to this belief. Is it hopeless?

 Reverse your statement, **I need me to** [*love*] _____ **and I need me to** [*love Me*] _____. Do you?

6. Read your statement. Repeat the usual steps.

 Now reverse it to **I am willing to** [*be like mother*] _____ or **I look forward to** [*being like mother*] _____.

 Repulsion is natural here, but you may as well look forward to it because you will think it again, which will bring you right back to The Work.

Once you have grasped the concept, a simpler way is to shift your perceptions from

I want him/her to . . .	to	**I want me to . . .**
He/she needs to . . .	to	**I need to . . .**
He/she should . . .	to	**I should . . .**
He/she is . . .	to	**I am . . .**
I don't want to . . .	to	**I look forward to . . .**

Remember, as each thought comes to you, to ask yourself, is it true, can I know that, what is the payoff for having this thought, who would I be without this belief?

A Personal Testimony

Witnesses to the value of The Work abound. One has already been mentioned in the case of Z, the gerontology specialist and consultant and daughter of a toxic ager. Near the end of chapter 5, Z expressed her gratitude to Katie and The Work for awakening her to the realization that much of her own personal pain and professional countertransference was caused, not by her mother's toxicity but by Z's perceptions of her mother and the consequential projections of Z's own toxicity onto her mother, an ego *defense mechanism* called projective identification.

Summary

Prevention of toxicity means self-help. It means a determined effort of persistent, self-disciplined inner work. As an anomaly of aging, toxicity can be stopped. With self-nourishment and love, those awakened to their susceptibility to toxicity can recognize early toxic patterns and their own stressors and can interrupt or break the generational cycle.

Candidates who can profit most from self-help, besides toxic-prone adult children (including professionals who are children of toxic agers), are older adults who fear becoming toxic and want to prevent it and early-stage toxic agers who recognize the symptoms and want to reverse the trend. The journey is not recommended for mentally or emotionally impaired older adults.

Case stories, a personal testimony, a scenario, and exercises illustrate the five areas of self-help: self-nourishment, stress management, stress reduction, support groups, and special programs.

Found in each category are some traditional techniques, such as self-affirmations; love notes; dance and quiet times; meditation; the Relaxation Response; negative self-talk reversal; deep breathing; assertion skills of Time Out, Stroke and Stand, Broken Record, Fogging, and I Messages; TA game stopping; and support groups and networks.

Also found in each category are unique and creative strategies, such as Target Strokes; warm fuzzies; personal Me Time; Mirror Talk; dialoguing within journaling; SUDS, a way to measure stress levels; and a challenging, special program exercise called The Work.

Chapter 14

The Path to Healing

*God has not given us
the spirit of fear.*

*God has given us
the spirit of
power
love
and a sound mind.*

II Timothy 1:7

Case Study

"D" is 62 years old. She is toxic and does not know it. A cure is inconceivable, but is healing possible?

Let us begin by recalling D's story, told to me through the pronounced pain in her voice. The time is the Great Depression. D was a small, only child when her mother died. D's father, a salesman and gambler, took D to live with one of her aunts, her uncle, and grandmother. It was not a healthy environment. D called it one of "screaming adults." The aunt (X) was prone to violent verbal attacks in which her face became red and the veins popped out in her neck. Even today, D replays her Jewish grandmother's warning, "Don't get X upset. She'll pop a blood vessel and die." In fear, D ran away from the tirades. She was scared, nervous, and shy. Her safety, she thought, came from constant strivings to please and unquestioning compliance.

It was not long before D's uncle died. He had been ill the entire 14 years he and X lived together. Then the grandmother died. They both died of colitis. D herself had stomach pains throughout the time she spent with X. Even as she talked about it, she felt the pains coming back.

D married, had three children, and moved as far away as she could, to California. Eventually, her two aunts (X and Y) followed. When Y's daughter deserted Y, D started to spend time with Y, taking her shopping and to the doctor. It was then, D said, "I learned a lot." Still, nothing changed.

D's father also followed to California, moving in temporarily with X until he could find a place to live. Soon he was at D's house every day, crying "She's killing me! She's killing me." Before he was able to move out, he died suddenly of an aneurysm.

It was not long before Aunt X started dropping in on D every day. Despite all the negative past experiences, D said nothing. After all, people kept telling her how wonderful her aunt was and how much she must love D. At least that was the way it appeared to the outside world. X was charming in public. She fooled everyone, including her lawyers. So D, with her lack of self-love, worth, and esteem, believed what outsiders told her. There must be something wrong with her.

Soon D's husband said he had had it with X dropping in all the time. He moved out, divorced D, and left her with three young children and no money.

D obtained a real-estate job and managed for a while until, as she tells it, the children grew and succumbed to their father's threats. He refused to give them any money if they had anything to do with their mother. With bitterness in her voice, D bewailed,

He turned the children against me. I've lost them for ever! They'll never come back!

By now D was having severe panic attacks and was diagnosed with agoraphobia. She lost everything, along with her job and her house. Aunt X again stepped in, telling D to come and live with her in a senior complex. They would share the home equally.

Desperate, D moved in. Later she discovered that X was telling D's children, "Your mother doesn't work. She just lies around." It seemed that D's illnesses included arthritis, knee problems, and a separation of the retina in her eye. D exclaimed,

I was forced to bed, the pain was so bad. X just makes it worse. She's always doing something to make me miserable, like the day she cleaned my room with ammonia and Clorox and then left, leaving me stuck in bed. And then there was another day. I was in bed, and X came in and screamed, 'What are you doing to me? Why don't you die already?'

Bemoaning her fate, D went on to proclaim,

X is living off, of dead people. She kills them off, then confiscates their money and belongings. She's already told my children they can have my Steinway piano. And the $35,000 trust in bonds that she set up for me when I was young; she helped my son cash them and took the money.

D went on to say that at one time, when things got so bad, she asked her aunt,

Why are you doing this to me? I'm the only person that ever loved you!

According to D, X only screamed back,

Love! What's love got to do with it?

Continuing, D said that X watched people until she found their weak points, then struck, pushing their buttons. X did this to a male friend of D's, who at first did not believe everything D was telling him about X. Finally one day, X got to D's friend. He apparently became defensive with X's criticisms and demeaning comments and "lost it," as D put it. It was then that he finally believed D and talked her into leaving. D went to stay with a friend.

Today, D says she is embarrassed to even talk about her situation and background. She laments,

No one in my family ever talks about feelings. And then to realize I'm 62, and just waking up to what my Aunt is! Maybe the countersuit I filed against her and my son will bring some resolution . . . (the pause is short) but I doubt I'll make it through the lawsuit. My stomach is already hurting.

(By the way, X is 93, trim, fit, and full of energy!)

Case Analysis

Can D be healed? Can X be healed? Study the case, reflect on it, then ask yourself the following:

- Who's toxic in this story and practicing woundology? What is the evidence, the signs and signals?
- Is there game playing? If so, what is the degree?
- Identify and name the games.
- How does the case connect with this book's premise that we respond to people or things according to the way we perceive them?
- Is there projection? Is projection perception? Explain what these mean.
- Can I discern the needs of D, of X? Describe them.
- What parts do fear, control, and responsibility play?

Much can be learned from this case. Recognize that few people realize how poisonous the toxins of toxicity can be. In its extreme state, as seen in X, toxicity can consume the co-Victim if he or she is vulnerable enough to permit its full impact, as seen with D.

With this case, it is tempting to agree with psychiatrist Scott Peck (1983) when he stated that there was evil in all humans, especially in ordinary people. As Peck defines it, "evil is that force, residing either inside or outside of human beings, that seeks to kill life or liveliness" (p. 43). "It will contaminate or otherwise destroy a person who remains too long in its presence" (p. 65). In essence, it consumes the spirit.

Peck further says people, noxious ones like X, sense there is something in their nature that is too fearful to acknowledge. They flee from its power, unconsciously projecting its energy outward onto others. It is a behavior that develops with use, occurring as people lie to themselves about who they are and what they feel and think. These people deny and disown parts of themselves, parts called the dark side of human nature, and if not embraced and tamed, they can unconsciously emerge with destructive results.

Review

D's story is a vivid example of how toxicity is passed on to the next generation. It also portrays what happens when there is a hole in the developmental process; when there is no demonstration of love, trust, and nourishment; and when there is no awareness of one's own distorted self-perceptions and how they in turn determine where one turns for love. D is not cognizant that, as a grown woman, it is her own lack of self-value, self-love, and self-respect that keeps her vulnerable to toxic games. For her, these are personal attributes that never had a chance to develop. Is D a victim or a Victim*?

Children, like D, are constantly seeking approval and attempting to please. They are desperate for some sense of worth, recognition, and control. In an environment such as the one in which D found herself, efforts to please and get positive strokes are futile. True love, the spiritual kind, is only found from within, not from outside sources. Such sources cannot heal the ego's fears or integrate the shadow.

Obviously, children raised in this type of toxic environment will model what they see and know. They can be excused for their behavior. As adults, however, rationalizations are no recourse. Adults have choices, not excuses. They can interrupt the syndrome. They can set boundaries and limits. They can break the generational cycle. They can build their self-esteem and manage their distress. They can learn to love and value themselves and others. Nobody, however, said it would be easy.

Transitioning

All of us are born both human and spirit, born into a worldly place possessing unique, individual personality traits that can be enhanced or crushed by environmental conditioning. There is much to learn. Guidance takes time. From our early teachers (significant others), we perceive messages of how we should be. We observe and we model. Then we write our own life script.

Few specifics are included on healthy ways to be or on how to take care of ourselves. Our interpretations of these teachings are, too often, distorted and flawed. It is no wonder that we build illusions of what we think we ought to be, what someone directed us to be, or what we imagine ourselves to be. Then our ego jumps in to help us defend our perceived choices. We become fixated. We do not, generally, prepare ourselves to reclaim that which we truly are. The journey toward our true Self is too hard, too fearful.

Instead, we hold onto indoctrinated attitudes, beliefs, and values from childhood. If they are toxic, we victimize ourselves. We imprison ourselves with fear, unable to break out, only to have our aliveness, our Self, suppressed.

Too often we are like the person in Plato's story of the Cave.

> A man was imprisoned in a dungeon. His only light came through one tiny crevice for a short time each day when the sun was at its peak. Even his food and water were passed to him in utter darkness. Each day the man would look forward to this brief period of time during which he would press close to the crevice so that he might catch a glimpse of some tiny part of the outside world. Then he would resign himself to total darkness until the next day. At first the man tried to explore his surroundings by feeling along the walls of the dungeon. When he discovered he was imprisoned in a cavernous area, he became afraid that, if he wandered too far, he would not be able to find his way back to the spot where this precious ray of light shone through each day. He never discovered that at the far end of the dungeon was an unlocked door leading to freedom. (Greenwald, 1977, p. viii)

Wellness and Holistic Health

Probably the best place to start on our path to freedom and healing is with our own self. It is that familiar place where we can begin to take charge of our life. We can begin to make healthful decisions. It is a place where we can choose a path of self-disciplined wellness practices. What is the task? It is to work toward becoming physically, socially, mentally, and emotionally whole and to prepare for the journey away from toxicity toward our true essence and unconditional love, the spiritual journey toward the Self.

What Is Wellness?

Wellness is a comprehensive, all-inclusive, holistic health program. When the word "practices" is added, it simply means a commitment to a daily effort of practicing all the component parts of wellness. My definition does not limit itself to physical fitness and nutrition programs. It attempts to unify all aspects of the mind, body, and spirit. In that sense, we can say that wellness is "the art of self-nourishment." It incorporates a multitude of practices that enhance individual wholeness and prevents toxicity.

Some years ago, I designed an information sheet that I called "Wellness Practices." Its focus is on lifestyle, how we live on a daily basis. Its theme is responsibility. Wellness, holistic healthy living, and self-nourishment are choices—ours. Prevention is cheaper than treatment is and more effective than intervention is. Prevention, however, takes self-discipline, remembered behavior. It takes a commitment. The question is, are we willing to make that commitment? Are we, as professionals, adult children, and older adults, willing to follow through in order to prevent our own toxicity and enable us to help clients, students, friends, and children prevent their toxicity?

The questions to ask are as follows:

- How well do my daily routine, my automatic thoughts, and my ingrained habits enhance my joy of living and my effectiveness as a professional, caregiver, adult child of a toxic ager, or older adult?
- How self-nourishing are my wellness practices?
- Am I disciplined enough to maintain these practices?
- How well do I cope and respond objectively and effectively to the dysfunctional lifestyles around me?
- How protective is my nourishment armor in inhibiting toxic contamination?
- How often do I do a self-check?

Now examine the following definition before you study and apply the list of Wellness Practices. For some of you this definition may be slightly different. It does not matter. My hope is that together we can inspire successful aging by establishing healthy perceptions and environments that will prevent the negative energy of toxicity from continuing to infiltrate the aging process.

Wellness Definition

Wellness is *not* just the absence of disease . . . it is much more. Wellness is a state of being; a goal; a wholeness of body, mind, and spirit; a process of well-being. It means a commitment to personal responsibility, disciplined choices, and a productive lifestyle. It means maintaining good care of our bodies through exercise and nutrition. It means using our minds constructively and expressing our emotions effectively and appropriately. It means being willing to creatively enhance our social, psychological, and spiritual growth in order to transform our levels of consciousness. It means to accept and appreciate ourselves and others, to look for (and see) the energy of divine love, beauty, and uniqueness in all that we encounter. It means experiencing the healing power of unconditional love and thus inner peace.

Wellness Practices

Use this guide to prevent medical and emotional problems and to promote new life patterns, rooted habits, informed choices, and self-pacing.

Hans Selye, originator of the word and concept of stress, had a code he lived by.

Go at your own pace, practice altruistic egoism, and earn your neighbor's love.

TABLE 14.1 Wellness Practices Chart

- Eat a balanced, high-nutrient-dense, low-stress, varied *diet* of fresh vegetables, fruit, low in fat, high in fiber, and complex carbohydrates. **NO** junk snacking.
- Curtail sugar, refined flour, salt, and *processed foods* such as those that are pickled and smoked, and sausages, hot dogs, and bacon.

- *Exercise* 10 to 20 minutes daily with a choice, or combination of, calisthenics, stretching, walking, yoga, and sport games. Use stairs instead of elevators, and park at the end of parking lots and walk. Quality is more important than quantity.
- Better yet, add 20 minutes of *aerobics*, 3 to 5 times a week for cardiovascular conditioning. Get your heart pumping at your personal target rate (220 minus age, times 75% of the balance) by stationary cycling, swimming, fast walking, bicycling, jazz exercise, and (jogging?).
- No *smoking*.
- Limit *caffeine* (coffee, soft drinks, excesses).
- Monitor alcohol, avoid *chemical substances*.
- Maintain *body fat* at 15% to 17% for men and 19% to 21% for women (more critical than weight measure). Pinch test is helpful. Two inches or more means excess fat.
- Relax or meditate regularly to *quiet the mind* and body. Make time to be alone, to focus, to center, to pray, to be open. Appreciate the sunset or sunrise, flowers, trees, birds, clouds, breezes, and so on, or try some aikido or tai chi.
- Get 6 to 8 hours of *sleep* daily, per personal need.
- Activate your *spiritual faith*, listen to an inner guide—a divine consciousness or universal energy force of unconditional love.
- *Resolve* anger and fear daily, then let it go.
- *Laugh* freely, especially at yourself. Have fun with little things, be spontaneous, avoid being grumpy.
- Develop and maintain a social *support network*. Friends can be good medicine.
- Manage and schedule *time* according to your own values, needs, and interests, not someone else's.
- Seek and get your daily *skin quotient*. At least four hugs a day or 10 minutes cuddling a furry pet. Use the healing stimulant of touch.
- Exercise *"Winner" thinking*. Practice positive self-talk and affirmations to restructure any negative thoughts, attitudes, and belief system.
- Whenever possible, give yourself, and others, daily *warm fuzzies*. Ask for specific unconditional strokes when needed. Contract with those close to you for your unique *target strokes*.
- Identify your internal and external *stressors*, games, or whatever you allow to get to you or hook you. Experiment with, and implement, creative new strategies for coping and shifting your perceptions.
- Accept the responsibility for your own *perceptions*, thinking, and choices. Be a beneficial presence and light wherever you are, in service and love.

The Journey Continues

Healing, as indicated by Selye, means more than just working on ourselves. It means reaching out and not tolerating the personal and collective thinking that discharges negative energy. It means recognizing that the toxicity prevalent in our societal systems today is pervasively contagious. It means that the inner awakening is only the start of the process, the jolting shake-up and revamping of the old self, the old systems. It means an acceptance and integration of our dark side, our personal and collective shadows, in order to become whole. It means no longer pretending to be what we are not. It means living the truth and integrating the polarities, both positive and negative, so that the negative no longer has unconscious control. It means changing both our inner and our outer systems. It means finding our true selves and learning how to love them, unconditionally. Can we do it?

Finding the Self

Erikson and Feil called it developing Integrity. For Jung, it was balancing the polarities. For The Course it is removing the blocks to love's presence. For the Enneagram it is transforming self-defeating behavior. Finding the Self has been the human search for wholeness from ancient times to today. It is an integration process that embraces and unifies the positive and the negative parts of us, the parts we disown, deny, and refuse to acknowledge. Jung called them the Shadow.

Embracing the Shadow

Shadows can be light or dark. Either way, they are the parts seen by the outside world, rarely by us. They are primitive, unrefined, animalistic, instinctive collections of impulses and reactions. If they are from the dark side, they are so shocking and appalling that we are compelled to keep the lid on in order to control and hide them from ourselves, and wishfully from others.

If the shadows are golden (the light side) but unacceptable in the early childhood environment and not allowed to flourish, as with toxics, it is our task to go deep inside and uncover them. They are often the undiscovered aptitudes and potentials that, if developed, may bring a new and exciting life full of joy, energy, meaning, and fulfillment when the old patterns no longer work.

According to Miller (1989, p. 93), Jung reminds us that

> Man is constantly inclined to forget that what was once good does not remain good eternally. He follows the old ways that once were good long after they have become bad, and only with the greatest sacrifices and untold suffering can he rid himself of this delusion and see that what was once good is now perhaps grown old and is good no longer.

Here Jung implies that what we once perceived as good was only the *ego* deluding us into believing we did not have to face ourselves. Stepping in with its advice and defenses, the ego temporarily resolves our doubts and fears. We compliantly build our illusions and a phoney self-image. It works for awhile.

Effort Needed

According to Gurdjieff, that illusion, that phoney self-image, can be penetrated only if we wake up. This awakening, this restoration of balance, can be as Jung said, of "greatest sacrifices and untold suffering." To Gurdjieff it requires a jolt powerful enough to shift our perceptions and transmute the negative disordered energy into positive emotional energy that will restructure and reorder the system. It is not an easy task.

Harry Moody, editor of *Aging and The Human Spirit* (1997), opened his editorial on "The Pursuit of Happiness" with "Why must I always act this way?" It was a comment blurted out in anger one day. It demonstrated the power of the unconscious shadow and its toxic dark side. It reinforced the difficulty in attempting to change oneself. According to Moody, "Many of us find ourselves acting out self-destructive patterns in life and in relationships with others without realizing what we are doing."

Moody wanted to escape his anger, but like most of us (especially toxics) he did not know how. Philosophizing, Moody referenced the Sufis, Muslim mystics who insist that abolishing anger could destroy its energy, and we could lose a "powerful ally on the Path." Buddhists also claim that paying attention to the dragon within, even if it terrorizes us, will remove it from our harm. It is our fear of ourselves that creates our suffering, not the truth. If we hold onto these fears, as do toxics, we only create more suffering.

Consequently, transcending the ego self, the self we mistakenly take ourselves to be, is our best option. Good intentions, self-help efforts, workshops, and psychotherapy are excellent preparations to cleanse some of the garbage and behavioral blocks, but none goes far enough. They are insufficient for the task of deep healing. Only Love can abolish fear. Letting go of ego defenses and their perceived protection, transcending the ego's power, is a journey so frightening it is almost impossible to travel without a spiritual guide. It requires a total integration of the body, mind, and spirit. It requires a faith surrender to Divine Grace and that healing power of Love.

Vignette

An example of the need for the spiritual component to healing is depicted in the answer Deepak Chopra gave to a professional in his newsletter (1997, October). The question was, "My mother makes me feel like a child. She always finds fault with my work, my relationships, and the amount of time I spend with her. What can I do?"

Chopra immediately focused on the professional's own need for approval and control as the reason she was being driven crazy, not on her mother. In essence, he told the daughter that until you can make a conscious choice to let go of the need to control and for approval, your emotions will build until they "create toxicity in your body and affect your health." Chopra recommended three steps:

1. Take responsibility for your own feelings.

2. Express them to yourself, possibly journaling.
3. Share your awareness with a loved one.

The jolt, the spiritual leap of transcending, of going beyond her frustration, anger, and ego comes with Chopra's last piece of advice. The loved one the professional was to share her feelings with was her mother.

Chopra (1997, October) continued,

> Assure [your mother] of your love and how important she is to you, and then share your whole experience with her. Never say, "You got me angry when . . . " Instead explain [using I messages], "This is what I felt every time I interacted with you, and I finally decided to deal with it. I realize these are my feelings and not your fault. I have now gone through this process, and because I love you so much, I want to share it with you."

There was no follow-up on the story, but without a spiritual faith and guide, it is doubtful that the daughter (even as a professional) would have been able to resist the power of the ego and the emotional glue that holds her imprisoned. It is even doubtful that she could pull out enough love for both herself and her mother to face the encounter.

The ego controls through fear, the highest level of energy acting on us, according to Richard Moss as expressed in a 1986 workshop I attended. It is that fear that the Child inside feels, an energy more powerful than logic or reason. Practice, such as behavioral rehearsal, can help the daughter face the expected conflict, even reduce her SUDS level, but will not reduce the deep feelings of fear and blame. Only unconditional love has the power to free her from her own self-inflicting suffering.

Reinforcement of Concept

Chopra's challenge to the professional daughter may sound extreme and even unreasonable, but emotional struggle is frequently experienced in spiritual growth and healing. In *A Course in Miracles* (1975), it is reiterated over and over that retraining the mind and being aware of the ego and its deceptively manipulative ability to jump in with quick fixes and defenses are only the first steps in clearing the garbage. They do not remove, however, the deep unconscious blocks to love nor open the door—that we have shut—to its healing power.

To truly awaken from our human condition requires more. It means a total shift in perception through unconditional acceptance, forgiveness, and love: a forgiveness of the self as well as the toxic, of not only what was done to us but also what was not done. It means the kind of perceptual shift the daughter in the vignette had to make in order to see her mother not as a toxic irritant but as a projection of the daughter's own self. It means the ability of the daughter to discern the love in her mother and to bring forth a different response pattern. It means sustaining a strength that is almost impossible unless manifested from within, at a deep spiritual level.

The Struggle

The struggle against toxicity is an individual one, always against our own fears, hurts, guilt, shadows, and the ego's hold. This struggle is against our own driven compulsions, personality tendencies, and environmental conditioning. It is against the ego's demand to continue to feed the inner monsters that seduce us into believing we are weak, frightened, and alone, unable to love and be loved.

We can control how we choose to respond to outside stimuli. We can decide whether to reject or allow it to control us. Final transformation and healing, however, are beyond our human frailties. That takes a Higher Power.

The Enneagram's Role

In my 40 years of experience in the human services field, the Enneagram (see chapter 8) was the first inclusive system that I found to embody the psychosocial, mental, and spiritual components as well as Eastern and Western thinking, thus my bias.

Especially effective is the map the Enneagram offers for the preparatory first part of the wholeness journey. By following the symbol's arrows, each personality type has a particular path to traverse in order to uncover its shadow and move to a higher, more healthy developmental level.

The journey may take a lifetime. Discomfort is a common companion. In addition, an inner spiritual guide is essential for avoiding the seductions of the ego and to prevent being mired in dysfunctional defenses, compulsions, and other ego-based fixations. No change will occur if the traveler stays on a cognitive or behavioral level only. Since truth is the ultimate desire, there is no other option but to move into the affective and deeper level of the soul and, as Gurdjieff propounds, jolt the system.

Apparently Eric Hoffer agreed when he said

> To dispose a soul to action, we must upset its equilibrium.

Upsetting the System

Disrupting ingrained thinking is part of the genius of the Enneagram. If individuals are ready, it can be a formidable, but complex, in-depth tool for identifying, owning, and integrating the shadow parts of us that we have refused to acknowledge or accept. As Hurley and Dobson (1991) proclaim, the Enneagram awakens us to our self-defeating attitudes, negative behaviors, and addictive compulsions. It also helps us to see how our weaknesses can be our strengths, if we but perceive these weaknesses differently. We can view them as gifts, as opportunities for growth. We can reframe negative behavior into acts of love, brought into being to teach us the perfect lesson we need to learn at that moment, and thus begin to dismantle the ego's power and entrapments.

It is in this framework that I especially see the connection between the Enneagram and toxicity. The Enneagram can be a valuable means for interrupting many lifelong, toxic patterns before they become destructive.

Besides interrupting addictive compulsions, the Enneagram can be used to uncover the more deeply constructed realities of the unhealthy, pathological lower self, a concept developed by

Don Riso in his original book, *Personality Types* (1987), which he expanded in his subsequent book *Understanding the Enneagram* (1990), and in the revised *Personality Types* (1996) with Russ Hudson. Riso established three categories (Healthy, Average, and Unhealthy) that identify where any of us, a client, or a co-Victim family member may be functioning.

Often when older adults are found in the Unhealthy, lower-self category, it is because they cannot, or will not, face the truth about themselves. The fear of the emotional consequences is just too painful. By the time we are old (or even adolescent old), we agers have learned countless ways to hide from what we do not want to know or do. We stay stuck in our negative energies and consciousness, blind to our own reality. Even when we are children, our egos con us into thinking we can maintain our self-illusions. Unfortunately, for the first half of life it generally works.

By the time older adulthood is reached the addiction to the unhealthy strategy of our particular Enneagram type is ingrained. Behavior is automatic. It is a ritualistic routine of deceit that goes on daily and becomes our identity. Any change of the familiar is resisted. Besides, even if we are toxic, the behavior yields recognition and negative strokes. It maintains the illusion. Why give it up? Addicts do not. They just need more negative strokes!

Healing—the Journey's End

To be healed is to be free, to be at inner peace, to transcend the human ego free of its addictive control, free of fear, and free to rest the spiritual sickness, the emptiness. It is worth the journey.

It is the third level of the Enneagram, the spiritual level, where we stop striving, surrender to our Higher Self, our true essence, and are open to a faith that believes the power of love can accomplish anything. It is a potent medicine, a mystery, yet, to attain it, we need do nothing more. Cleansing the garbage has been accomplished. The blocks to love have been removed. We can observe ourselves with detachment and acceptance. We are beyond fear. We are open to Divine Grace.

We no longer need the payoffs of Victimization. We no longer feel fragmented, separate from others and our Creator. We no longer usurp His or Her role. Guilt and anger are gone. Perceptions and responses have shifted; we have dropped the script, the games, and our false self. We know we are loved and can love. We know we *are* Love.

Summary

This chapter opens with the story of two older women: an old-old advanced and extreme case of toxicity and a young-old co-Victim. Each is toxic. Each has her own inner demons. The questions are

- Is healing possible?
- Can they travel the path to get there?

To consider these questions, the chapter focuses on the paths to healing and the transformational process. It begins with recognizing healing as different from curing. Healing is holistic and encompasses all parts of us: the body, the mind, and the spirit. It embodies the physical, mental, social, emotional, and spiritual aspects of who we are. It recognizes that we cannot heal ourselves, but we can prepare for the journey in order to be open and ready for the healing mystery.

The start is a commitment, a choice to sustain self-efforts such as those exemplified in the list of daily, holistic health, personal wellness practices. Combined with total emergence in self-development workshops, systems such as the Enneagram, and persistence, it is possible to travel the path toward healing and eventually open the door to the unknown. With these efforts and final ego release, the false self personality and dark side shadow are awakened and brought into the light. Self-defeating behavior, guilt, fear, and other blocks to Love are cleansed. Fragments of self, the disowned shadow, are integrated. Projections stop, self-love is accepted and practiced, and the toxic within, with its perceived benefits, is rejected.

Yet, the journey is still not complete. The above is only the path. The remainder of the healing journey is beyond our control.

It is a letting go, a surrendering to a Higher Self, to a Divine Presence. It is a releasing of all fear and movement into unquestioning faith.

It may not mean a medical or physical cure. It does, however, mean freedom and inner peace. It means no longer having to please or be in control, no longer being afraid of being vulnerable, no longer in emotional, physical, mental, social, or spiritual pain. It means being loved unconditionally because we are Love. We are a presence, and everyone we touch will know that Love. *That* is healing.

Is it possible? You decide.

Afterword

Although this book was designed and written for professionals in the gerontology field, my dream is that everyone reading it will see the need to start the process of toxicity prevention relative to future agers and generational passage plus make certain that older adults who are already toxic are surrounded by steadfast boundaries of unconditional love.

Does that mean pity? Trying to please? Distancing?

No! Surrounding toxic agers with steadfast boundaries and love means to BE there, to be a presence but detached and free from seductive toxic hooks and games. It means setting personal limits and boundaries. It means loving yourself enough to quell your own fears and defenses, enabling and empowering you to sustain objective support. It means being the catalyst, when appropriate and responsible, that jolts the toxic loop and, in a sense, spiritually forces toxic agers to reach for the love that is buried deep inside them, to struggle through the process of assuming responsibility for their own lives and to find and draw out their long-denied, inner resources. It means rejecting Victim consciousness.

Advice to the Aging

If you see yourself
as sour grape juice,
acidify you will.

If you see yourself
as vintage wine,
mellow you will be.

—gloria d.

Glossary[*]

Adapt — to fit in, to adjust to one's environment, to settle, to make comfortable, to bring to a proper position, to flow with what is.

Addiction — an Enneagram term used by Hurley and Dobson to mean the same as the ego-fixation or compulsion. A habitual pattern, unconsciously controlled by our shadow that compels us to act contrary to our conscious values or logical mind. A sense of negative, destructive comfort when acted on.

Agers — those who are aging, here referring to individuals 65 years of age or older. (See Old Old for aging classifications.)

Aging — a continual process of adaptive response patterns that interact with both internal and external forces across time and enhance, modify, or change productivity capabilities.

Anomaly — deviation from norm, type, or form; irregularity.

Beingness — a term used to denote being the whole Self, unfettered by illusions, roles, the persona, or false image or mask.

[*]Defined in accord with use in this text.

Care Providers — different from caregivers; particularly referring to adult children who do not give direct care but take on the responsibility for overseeing the continued well-being and financial needs of an aging parent.

Character — a distinguishing feature or attribute of integrity and strength, a moral or ethical structure of a person or group.

Construct — a process or act of creating, devising, forming or structuring; of integrating or putting together divergent parts; or to set in order based on one's perceptual interpretation.

Countertransference — a professional's unconscious overreaction to situations reminiscent of earlier relationships, positive or negative. Usually taps into difficult past experiences that cause the reliving of felt anxiety, revulsion, fearfulness, irritation, overprotection or underprotection, or other emotional pain. (Self-observation is especially crucial here if also an adult child of a toxic ager.)

Co-Victims — a collaboration of self-righteous sufferers who unconsciously play the Victim role in psychological game playing.

Cybernetics — an attempt to formulate a universal, unifying system to explain life. A key component: the closed feedback loop system.

Defense Mechanisms — according to the DSM-IV (APA, 1994, p. 765), defense mechanisms are an "automatic psychological process that protects the ego against anxiety and from awareness of internal or external stressors or dangers. Defense mechanisms mediate the individual's reaction to emotional conflicts," thus helping him or her to maintain an illusionary self-image, persona, or false self, and avoid facing, owning, and dealing responsibly with his or her own behavior.

Some mechanisms such as projection and acting out are "almost invariably maladaptive, whereas others such as repression and denial may be either maladaptive or adaptive, depending on their severity, their inflexibility, and the context in which they occur" (APA, 1994, p. 765).

The following are some of the specific defense mechanisms used by toxic agers to deal with emotional conflict or internal or external stressors as described primarily by the DSM-IV (APA, 1994, pp. 755–757).

Acting Out — deals with emotions by actions rather than reflections or feelings.

Denial — refusal to acknowledge or recognize some painful aspect of an external reality or subjective experience that would be apparent to others.

Displacement — transferring a feeling or response to a less-threatening object or person.

Emotional Insulation — avoidance of emotional pain or rejection, consciously controlling and repressing all feelings, never truly loving or showing vulnerableness.

Help-Rejecting Complaining — making repetitious requests for help that disguise covert feelings of hostility or reproach toward others that are then expressed by rejecting the suggestions, advice, or help offered. (In TA terms known as the "Yes, but" game.)

Isolation of Affect — separation of ideas or cognitions from the feelings originally associated with them, for example, a traumatic event.

Passive Aggression — indirectly and unassertively expressing aggression toward another. A facade of overt compliance covering covert resistance, resentment, or hostility.

Projection — falsely attributing to another one's own unacceptable feelings, impulses, or thoughts in order to justify the discounts and criticisms placed on the other for then having those traits. With these deceptive projections, one does not have to deal with, or own, his or her own behavioral flaws.

Projective Identification — same as projection, but uses the projections to justify own impulses and affect. Can induce these very feelings in others, making it difficult to discern who did what to whom.

Rationalization — making excuses or self-serving elaborations to conceal true motivations and avoid facing intolerable situations or reality, for example, if feeling hurt one would say "Oh, it's OK, it doesn't matter," or "I prefer being alone," or "I don't like them either."

Reaction Formation — substituting behavior, thoughts, or feelings that are totally opposite of own unacceptable thoughts, behavior, or feelings, such as smiling sweetly to toxic agers. (Usually in conjunction with repression.)

Repression — the expulsion of disturbing, unacceptable wishes, thoughts, or experiences from conscious awareness. Feelings may remain conscious but disassociated and detached.

Degree — a Transactional Analysis term used to differentiate three levels of game playing that substitute for genuine interpersonal transactions. First degree: socially acceptable. Second degree: concealed from the public. Third degree: played for keeps: tissue or psychic damage, or both (Berne, 1964, p. 64). Toxics are skilled at all levels.

Developmentally Fixated — a term coined by author to indicate a fixation or being stuck, at an Eriksonian stage of development. In reference to toxics, it would be the first stage: trust.

Dis-ease — a New Age, wholistic health term used to connote more than a biophysical condition but a combination of distress-inducing situations that yield psychosocial-physical ramifications.

DSM-IV — *Diagnostic and Statistical Manual of Mental Disorders* (1994). Produced by the American Psychiatric Association as their basic diagnostic resource tool.

Ego — based on fear, it is the human subconscious force within the mind that is the executor of the personality or false self-illusions. It protects its power base by deceptively manipulating and controlling thoughts, responses, and subsequent external behavior (see Defense mechanisms).

Ego-Fixation — term used by Ichazo to designate the point in the Enneagram where a person is stuck in a compulsed ego defense position.

Ego States — structural analysis component of Transactional Analysis. Diagrammatically formed in three circles.

Emotional Deprivation — a term coined by R. Spitz to denote an irreversible decline and proneness to disease in institutionalized infants if deprived of social and sensory handling and emotional support over a long period of time.

Extraversion — a Jungian term meaning that energy is attained by going outside the person, usually in conjunction with other people.

Frustration — a deep chronic sense or state of insecurity and dissatisfaction arising from unresolved problems or unfulfilled needs.

Games — unconscious, psychological transactions, played indefinitely by two people if they know the rules and have a hidden agenda. Game playing is recognized by the bad-feeling payoff at the end. Named by Transactional Analysis founder Eric Berne, there are three levels of games (see Degree). Advanced toxics operate at the third-degree level.

Gerontophilia — extreme form of positive ageism or excessive love of aging and elders (Palmore, 1990, p. 38).

Gerontophobia — extreme form of negative ageism or an "unreasonable fear and/or irrational hatred of older people" (Bunzel, 1972).

Healing — in this definition, to heal is not synonymous with the body or the medical term cure. Healing is much broader. It encompasses the whole person—the integration of the physical, mental, social, emotional, and spiritual into a total sense of wholeness, peace, well-being, and transcendence. In this context a person may physically die but still be healed.

Help-Rejecting Complaining — incessant complaining about offered services, with no intention of compliance.

Hooked — a term used in Transactional Analysis to designate when individuals allow themselves to be caught, or "taken in," by the playing of a psychological game.

Integrate — to make whole, to bring together all aspects or parts, to join, to unify, to unite.

Integrity — state of being complete, undivided, unbroken or whole; of accepting, owning, and realistically integrating and balancing the tensions between opposing parts of self, plus reintegrating the psychosocial stages of life development.

Introversion — a Jungian term for restoring personal energy by going within. Attained by Introverts through withdrawal and private space.

Irritate — to provoke impatience, anger, or displeasure in; implies an often gradual arousing of angry feelings that may range from mere impatience to rage.

Karpman's Triangle — an inverted triangle that designates the interactive points of a psychological game in Transactional Analysis. The points are known as Victim, Persecutor, and Rescuer.

Life Script — A Transactional Analysis term that likens a script of life to a theater play. The author is the child between 2 and 7 years of age who subconsciously writes the script according to how messages from significant others are perceived, then selects the cast and the staging to carry out the plot.

Maladaptive — a psychological term for an inability to adapt to the normal demands of life; to adjust to the environment, transitions, and relationships; and, in aging, to maximize and balance integrity and productivity.

Negative Energy — a capacity for action or power in the form of a deconstructive force or direction.

Neurosis — a term popularized by Karen Horney in the late 1930s implying a disturbance of the personality and character structure whereby the individual is torn by inner emotional conflicts and relational problems yielding a psychic illness of undifferentiated origin.

Noxious — injurious to physical health and also harmful to the mind or morals; hurtful; causing or intending to cause damage; pernicious.

Old-Old — one of the three classifications used by researchers and academicians to designate the different levels of aging. Generally based on chronological age, they are roughly as follows:

Traditional	With my added fourth category
Young-Old: 55–64	Young-Old: 55–64
Old: 65–79	Adolescent-Old: 65–74
Old-Old: 80+	Old: 75–84
	Old-Old: 85+

Although each ager is unique and develops individually and at different rates, it is useful to know (as in child development) that there are different phases and task expectations at each level. Here are my perceptions:

Young-Old Task — to maintain or become fit, trying on new roles, uncovering hidden talents, living to the fullest.

Adolescent-Old Task — a period of exploration, experimentation, asking, and discovering "Who am I as an old person?"

Old Task — striving for integrity or wholeness, deepening spiritual beingness, finding the Self, and living fully with inner joy.

Old-Old Task — resolving old, unfinished issues and conflicts, beginning to disengage from life and achieving inner peace and oneness with God.

Passion — any intense, extreme, or overpowering emotion. In Enneagram terms it means the driving force (negative if in excess) of the ego characterization of each personality type.

Payoff — the Transactional Analysis bad feeling present at the end of every psychological game. Called a payoff because one of the reasons for playing games is to collect negative strokes that then become the payoff for playing.

Perceived Reality — that which exists as real in the mind of the perceiver whether factual or illusory.

Perception (psychosocial) — mental, image response patterns formed through the perception process.

Perceptual Process — a complex, multisensory series of spontaneous mental steps whereby individuals (often unconsciously) sort, organize, interpret, define, and construct their internal pictures of reality and subsequent lifestyle in interaction with incoming sensations, expectations, frame of reference, prior learning experiences, needs, values, belief systems, and social and cultural conditioning.

Perceptual Shift — term used to describe a tool for dealing with problem areas or breaking resistance to change. By shifting the perception from a negative outcome to a positive outcome or by seeing the person, thing, or irritant differently, the response can be reversed, personal power reclaimed, and control maintained. This means the problem can be shifted to a challenge and creatively solved.

Persecutor — always capitalized when used as part of Karpman's Triangle and a psychological game in Transactional Analysis.

Personality — the external false self and ego illusion that presents a predictable set of response patterns and styles of behavior. Formed by internal perceptions, it is constructed to make the self socially acceptable.

Productive — having the quality, ability, and personal power to produce, to generate results, or to bring forth in a positive manner.

Projection — See Defense mechanisms.

Psyche — the essence of the psychospiritually integrated whole; ostensibly the nonmaterial nature of humans including the mind, emotions, and soul.

Rescuer — otherwise known as the "Big R," also capitalized as part of Karpman's Triangle and a pitfall especially for new professionals if they are not watchful and aware of overcaring and making clients dependent.

Self — used by Jung with a capital to distinguish the balanced integrated Self, the true essence, from the personality self.

Self-perception — based on a self-perceptual process, a person's construct of self and personality style.

Shadow — term coined by Jung meaning the unknown, the hidden part of us (either positive or negative, golden or dark) that is primitive, archaic, infantile, disowned, unrecognized, unacknowledged, feared, and untamed. Can break out at any time.

Signals — a communicative indicator or sign that can trigger a specific response, action, or message.

Spiritual awakening — becoming the true Self, recognizing, owning, accepting, and integrating all parts, including addictions and compulsions. It is listening to the inner voice that refuses to be silenced by the incessant, self-serving demands and defenses of the ego.

Stress (also known as distress) — a physical, mental, or emotional strain and tension that is regarded as a threat to psychological and social well-being.

Stressor — an internal or external perception, force, or person that causes distress.

Strokes (Positive) — Transactional Analysis term referring to affirmations and behavior that are units of love or nourishment.

Successful Aging — according to gerontologist Jim Birren, it means "adapting to the demands made on us so as to maximize our productivity and integrity." This is exhibited by the ability to flow with life, maintain a healthy balance and meaningful lifestyle, be functionally independent, and have a positive attitude and worldview.

SUDS — abbreviation for "Successful Units of Discomfort Scale," a symbolic measure of optimal stress levels.

Tape — Transactional Analysis term denoting a computer-like recording in the brain of perceived early messages that determine future behavior and are relentlessly played in our heads until erased or overwritten.

Toxic — a negative energy state, or self-Victimizing consciousness and pattern of thinking, feeling, perceiving, and behaving that is poisonous to the self and anyone vulnerable to its toxins.

Advanced, or full-blown toxics possess a contagious behavior that drains, depresses, and depletes. Known as "Blamers," "Whiners," or "Bitchers," toxics are obsessed with their own pain. Torn by inner emotional conflict and a hateful self-perception, they cover their fears and guilt by projecting them onto others, called projective identification, one of many skillfully developed defense mechanisms.

Although also turned inward, toxicity is typically manifested in acting-out behavior consisting of persistent and excessive complaining, demanding, fault-finding, manipulative control, psychological game-playing, paranoia, self-pity, martyrdom, alienation, and self-deceit. Toxics do not know how to love and nourish themselves, ask for what they need, or express their feelings appropriately.

Toxic Agers — elderly adults who habitually exhibit the negative symptoms of toxicity.

Toxicity (Davenport's Psychological Definition) — a developmentally fixated, character maladaptation and life pattern of thinking, feeling, and perceiving that manifests in an obsessive negative energy of Victim consciousness and unaware controlling and compulsive behavior.

Toxicity in Agers — pervasive negative behaviors and attitudes that destructively impact social interactions. Toxic behavior tends to alienate professionals, family, and friends, often leading to social isolation of the toxic person. In extreme cases, toxicity can lead to the withdrawal of services and social supports by the very individuals that the toxic ager needs for assistance in maintaining effective functioning or independent living, or both.

Toxic Loop — an endlessly playing, feedback cycle of energy-draining responses and signals.

True Self — same as true essence; the person we were born to be; our psychosocial-spiritual whole.

Unsuccessful Aging — also referred to as toxic aging, a nonnormal, dysfunctional, Victimized perception and response pattern to life.

Very Successful Aging — includes all the components of Successful Aging plus an energy and zest for life, an active, involved lifestyle, a continuous effort to seek ways to grow, an eager desire to serve and contribute to the community, and an inspiring attitude or worldview.

Victim — specifically capitalized to signify one of the three roles played in Karpman's Triangle: an illustration of the dynamics of the psychological games of Transactional Analysis. The Victim is always at the bottom of the triangle, a position that implies suffering and victimization. If the term is not capitalized, it designates true victimization, not a game.

Victim Consciousness — a perception of self as having been abused by environmental forces that become the root of a self-imprisoning fear. This, in turn, gives the Victim permission to be a martyr, with justified self-pity and a sense of righteousness in blaming others, and the past, without responsibility for one's own actions.

Warm Fuzzies — positive unconditional strokes that are genuine and authentic and leave a person feeling good, warm, and loved.

Woundology — a term coined by Caroline Myss to represent a Victim consciousness mindset that asserts "when we define ourselves by our wounds, we burden and lose our physical and spiritual energy and open ourselves to the risk of illness (1997, p. 6). This self-induced focus and pity causes an energy leak that locks the Victim into the wound and blocks healing and transformation. When used as a pivotal point for endless sharing and commiseration, it becomes a misuse of self-expression and, unfortunately, is too often supported by like-minded groups and relationships, becoming a sanctioned power base for manipulating others.

References

A course in miracles. (1975). Tiburon, CA: Foundation for Inner Peace. Three books: text, student workbook, teachers manual.

American Psychiatric Association. (1968). *Diagnostic and statistical manual of mental disorders* (2nd ed.). Washington, DC: Author.

American Psychiatric Association. (1987). *Diagnostic and statistical manual of mental disorders* (3rd ed., rev.). Washington, DC: American Psychiatric Press.

American Psychiatric Association. (1994). *Diagnostic and statistical manual of mental disorders* (4th ed.). Washington, DC: American Psychiatric Press.

Aneshensel, C. S., Pearlin, L. I., Mullan, J. T., Zarit, S. H., & Whitlatch, C. J. (1995). *Profiles in caregiving: The unexpected career.* New York: Academic Press.

Atchley, R. C. (1972). *The social forces in later life.* Belmont, CA: Wadsworth Publishing.

Atchley, R. C. (1989). A continuity theory of normal aging. *Gerontologist, 29,* 183–190.

Baron, R., & Wagele, E. (1994). *The Enneagram made easy.* New York: HarperCollins.

Baron, R., & Wagele, E. (1995). *Are you my type, am I yours?* San Francisco: Harper.

Beesing, M., Nogosek, R. J., & O'Leary, P. H. (1984). *The Enneagram: A journey of self-discovery.* Denville, NJ: Dimension Books.

Berne, E. (1964). *Games people play.* New York: Ballantine Books.

Birren, J. E. (1987, April 24). *Spiritual maturity and psychological development.* Paper presented at the conference on "Aging and Wholeness in Later Years," Claremont School of Theology, Claremont, CA.

Birren, J. E., & Schaie, W. K. (1996). *Handbook of the psychology of aging* (4th ed.). New York: Academic Press.

Bowlby, J. (1969–1980). *Attachment and loss. Vol. 1: Attachment, Vol. 2: Separation: Anxiety and anger, Vol. 3: Loss: Sadness and depression.* New York: Basic Books.

Brady, L. (1994). *Beginning your Enneagram journey through self-observation.* Allen, TX: Tabor Publishing.

Bunzel, J. (1972). Note on the history of a concept—Gerontophobia. *Gerontologist, 12,* 116.

Chopra, D. (1997). *The path to love: Renewing the power of spirit in your life.* New York: Harmony Books.

Chopra, D. (1997, September). An interview with Candace Pert, Ph.D. re: Molecules in emotions. *Infinite Possibilities for Body, Mind, and Soul [Newsletter], 1*(12).

Chopra, D. (1997, October). Answering your questions. *Infinite Possibilities for Body, Mind, and Soul [Newsletter], 2*(1).

Cohler, B. J. (1991). Life course perspectives on the study of adversity, stress and coping: Discussion of papers from the West Virginia Conference. In E. M. Cummings, A. L. Green, & K. H. Karraker (Eds.), *Life-span developmental psychology: Perspectives on stress and coping* (pp. 297–326). Hillsdale, NJ: Erlbaum.

Covey, H. C. (1981). A reconceptualization of continuity theory: Some preliminary thoughts. *The Gerontologist, 21,* 628–633.

Davenport, G. M. (1991). *Determinants of successful aging.* Ann Arbor: University Microfilms International.

Dryer, P. (1985, Spring). *Development during old age.* Class lecture. Claremont, CA: Claremont Graduate School.

Erikson, E. H., Erikson, J. M., & Kivnick, H. Q. (1986). *Vital involvement in old age: The experience of old age in our time.* New York: Norton.

Evans, P. (1996). *The verbally abusive relationship: How to recognize it and how to respond.* Holbrook, MA: Adams Media Corporation.

Feil, N. (1992a). *VIF Validation: The Feil Method—How to help disoriented old-old.* Cleveland, OH: Feil Productions.

Feil, N. (1992b, March 27). *Validation Therapy Workshop.* Orange, CA. (For professionals in the aging field.)

Feil, N. (1997). *Myrna, the mal-oriented* [video]. Cleveland, OH: Edward Feil Productions.

Forward, S. (with Buck, C.). (1989). *Toxic parents: Overcoming their hurtful legacy and reclaiming your life.* New York: Bantam Books.

Forward, S. (with Frazier, D.). (1997). *Emotional blackmail: When the people in your life use fear, obligation and guilt to manipulate you.* New York: HarperCollins.

Gatz, M., Kasl-Godley, J. E., & Karel, M. J. (1996). Aging and mental disorders. In J. E. Birren & K. Schaie (Eds.), *Handbook of the psychology of aging* (4th ed., pp. 365–382). New York: Academic Press.

Glasser, W. (1981). *Stations of the mind: New directions for reality therapy.* New York: Harper & Row.

Glasser, W. (1985). *Control theory: A new direction for reality therapy.* New York: Harper & Row.

Greenwald, J. (1968). *The art of emotional nourishment.* Unpublished monograph.

Greenwald, J. (1969). *The art of emotional nourishment: Self-induced nourishment and toxicity.* Unpublished monograph.

Greenwald, J. (1973). *Be the person you were meant to be.* New York: Dell.

Greenwald, J. (1977). *Is this really what I want to do?* Pasadena: Ward Ritchie Press.

Harris, T. A. (1967). *I'm Ok—You're OK.* New York: Avon.

Hillman, J., & Ventura, M. (1992, June). Is therapy turning us into children? *New Age, 9*(3), 60–65, 136–141.

Horney, K. (1937). *The neurotic personality of our time.* New York: W. W. Norton.

Horney, K. (1992). *Our inner conflicts: A constructive theory of neurosis.* New York: W. W. Norton. (Original work published 1945.)

Hurley, K. V., & Dobson, T. E. (1991). *What's my type?—using the Enneagram system to identify the secret promise of your personality type, break out of your self-defeating patterns, & transform your weaknesses into unimagined strengths.* San Francisco: HarperCollins Publishers.

Hurley, K. V., & Dobson, T. E. (1993). *My best self: Using the Enneagram to free the soul.* San Francisco: HarperCollins.

Jakobowski, P., & Lange, A. J. (1979). *The assertive options.* Champaign, IL: Research Press.

James, M., & Jongeward, D. (1973). *Born to win.* Menlo Park, CA: Addison-Wesley.

Jerusalem Bible. (1966). Garden City, NY: Doubleday.

Johnson, S. (1997, September/October). The biology of love: What therapists need to know about attachment. *Family Therapy Networker, 21*(5), 37–41.

Jung, C. G. (1921). *Psychological types.* Princeton, NJ: Princeton University Press.

Katie, B. (1996). *What to do when nothing works.* Hopkins, MN: Sharpe Import Co.

Keyes, M. F. (1990). *Emotions and the Enneagram: Working through your shadow life script.* Muir Beach, CA: Molysdatur Publications.

Lange, A. J., & Jakobowski, P. (1976). *Responsible assertive behavior: Cognitive-behavioral procedures for trainers.* Champaign, IL: Research Press.

Love, P. (1990). *The emotional incest syndrome: What to do when a parent's love rules your life.* New York: Bantam Books.

Maltz, M. (1969). *Psycho-cybernetics.* New York: Prentice Hall.

McKay, M., Davis, M., & Fanning, P. (1981). *Thoughts and feelings.* Oakland, CA: New Harbinger Press.

Miller, A. (1990). *For your own good: Hidden cruelty in child-rearing and the roots of violence* (3rd ed.). New York: Noonday Press.

Miller, W. A. (1981). *Make friends with your shadow: How to accept and use positively the negative side of your personality.* Minneapolis, MN: Augsburg Fortress.

Miller, W. A. (1989). *Your golden shadow: Discovering and fulfilling your undeveloped self.* San Francisco: Harper & Row.

Milligan, M. J. (1997, June 9). *Issues of substance abuse and aging.* Report presented at a meeting of the Older Adults Services Committee, Orange County Mental Health Board of Behavioral Health Care, Santa Ana, CA.

Moody, H. R. (Ed.). (1997, Spring). Pursuit of happiness. *Aging and The Human Spirit Newsletter, 7*(1), 1, 2.

Moss, R. (1986). Self-development workshop. Lucerne Valley, CA.

Myss, C. (1996). *Anatomy of the spirit: The seven stages of power and healing.* New York: Harmony Books.

Myss, C. (1997). *Why people don't heal and how they can.* New York: Harmony Books.

Naranjo, C. (1997). *Transformation through insight: Enneatypes in life, literature, and clinical practice.* Prescott, AZ: Hohm Press.

Neugarten, B. L., Havighurst, R. J., & Tobin, S. S. (1968). Personality and patterns of aging. In B. L. Neugarten (Ed.), *Middle age and aging.* Chicago: University of Chicago Press.

Northrup, C. (1996, July). *Toxic emotions: Healing the symptoms they cause.* Potomac, MD: Phillips Publishing.

Ouspensky, P. D. (1949/1977). *In search of the miraculous.* San Diego, CA: Harcourt Brace Jovanovich.

Palmer, H. (1988). *The Enneagram: A definitive guide to the ancient system for understanding yourself and the others in your life.* San Francisco: Harper & Row.

Palmer, H. (1995). *The Enneagram: Exploring the nine psychological types and their inter-relationships in love and life* [Audiotape]. San Francisco: Harper.

Palmore, E. B. (1990). *Ageism negative and positive.* New York: Springer Publishing Co.

Peck, S. (1983). *People of the lie: The hope for healing human evil.* New York: Simon & Schuster.

Pert, C. (1997). *Molecules in emotions.* New York: Simon & Schuster.

Powers, W. T. (1973). *Behavior: The control of perception.* Chicago: Aldine.

Quenk, N. L. (1993). *Beside ourselves: Our hidden personality in everyday life.* Palo Alto, CA: CPP Books.

Reedy, M. N. (1983). Personality and aging. In D. S. Woodruff & J. E. Birren (Eds.), *Aging: Scientific perspectives and social issues* (pp. 112–121). Monterey, CA: Brooks, Cole.

Reichard, S., Livson, R., & Peterson, G. (1968). Adjustment to retirement. In B. L. Neugarten (Ed.), *Middle age and aging.* Chicago: University of Chicago Press.

Riordan, K. (1975). Gurdjieff. In C. T. Tart (Ed.), *Transpersonal psychologies.* New York: Harper & Row.

Riso, D. R. (1987). *Personality types.* Boston: Houghton Mifflin.

Riso, D. R. (1990). *Understanding the Enneagram.* Boston: Houghton Mifflin.

Riso, D. R., & Hudson, R. (1996). *Personality types: Understanding the Enneagram.* Boston: Houghton Mifflin.

Roberts, S. C. (1992). Multiple realities—How MPD is shaking up our notions of the self, the body and even the origins of evil. *Common Boundary: Between Spirituality and Psychotherapy, 10*(3), 24–31.

Rohr, R. (1995). *Enneagram II: Advancing spiritual discernment.* New York: Crossroad Publishing.

Ruth, J.-E., & Coleman, P. (1996). Personality and aging: Coping and management of the self in later life. In J. E. Birren & K. W. Schaie (Eds.), *Handbook of the psychology of aging* (4th ed., pp. 308–322). San Diego, CA: Academic Press.

Schlossberg, N. K. (1990). Training counselors to work with older adults. *Generations: Journal of the American Society on Aging, 14,* 7–10.

Secunda, V. (1990). *When you and your mother can't be friends: Resolving the most complicated relationship of your life.* New York: Delta Press.

Selye, H. (1975). *Stress without distress.* New York: Signet.

Spitz, R. (1945). Hospitalism: genesis of psychiatric conditions in early childhood. *Psychoanalytic Study of the Child, 1,* 53–74.

Steinbeck, J. (1962). *Travels with Charley.* New York: Viking.

Tart, C. (Ed.). (1983). *Transpersonal psychologies.* El Cerrito, CA: Psychological Processes.

Tart, C. T. (1986). *Waking up: Overcoming the obstacles to human potential.* Boston: New Science Library, Shambhala.

Turner, J. S., & Helms, D. B. (1979). *Life span development.* Philadelphia: W. B. Saunders.

U.S. Department of Commerce, Age and Sex Statistics Branch, Population Division, Bureau of the Census. (1993, September). *We the American . . . Elderly.* Washington, DC: U.S. Government Printing Office.

Index

Index